STICKS AND STONES

I0103332

By Lawrence Butterfield

chipmunkapublishing
the mental health publisher
empowering people with depression

Sticks and Stones

Published by
Chipmunkapublishing
PO Box 6872
Brentwood
Essex CM13 1ZT
United Kingdom

http://www.chipmunkapublishing.com

Edited by Aleksandra Lech

Chipmunkapublishing gratefully acknowledges the support of Arts Council England.

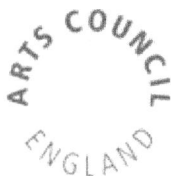

Sticks and Stones

The names of three patients mentioned 30 years ago have been changed to protect anonymity.

Sticks and Stones

"For those without a voice"

Sticks and Stones

Sticks and Stones

ACKNOWLEDGEMENTS

There are so many people I would like to thank
that if I named them all individually I would
probably fill another book. My family, colleagues,
patients, friends, in a career in Mental Health
Services that has touched almost 30 years. I
would though like to mention a few people and by
doing this I hope that others wouldn't feel too
offended by being left out. This is not my intention.

Thanks go to Jason Pegler, Andrew Latchford, and
Mary Dow from Chipmunkapublishing for giving
me the opportunity to write this book and all the
support given. Ben Furner, Sue Flook and Tertia
Cornet for their support, friendship, and expertise
ensuring my SHIFT Speakers Bureau work goes
smoothly. Always on the end of the phone, and
nothing is ever too much trouble. Teresa, my wife
for still tolerating me after 29 years, and my
children Steven and Laura, I am proud of you both
and always will be. My gratitude also goes to
Marjorie Wilson for her creative mind, her vision,
and inspirational approach to the "Huge Bag of
Worries" project. Both Marie Levy and Marie
Turbill from the Evening Gazette, who have
supported my newspaper articles, thereby helping
to deliver the anti stigma message through the
local newspaper. I appreciate their
acknowledgement of the importance of positively
profiling mental health issues through the press
and having the foresight to allow me to have a
dedicated column to spread the word. Jeanette

Sticks and Stones

Duffy, Simon Clayton, Caroline Parnell, John Kerr, Gemma Gray and Tees, Esk & Wear Valleys NHS Foundation Trust who have all supported me over the past 6 years in my work through the "Passionate People" campaign, some of whom have now left and moved to new roles. Simon Punton and Janice Collins my Line Managers from within the Trust I work for; without their support I would not be able to do this work, which can be challenging within a busy clinical area with patients to support. Ian Holliday and Mary Mohan from Redcar and Cleveland Social Services who have provided the time and support for me to continue with this work through a part time seconded role. On a more personal level Barry Hudson for being an excellent role model/mentor for me when working on the wards, and "Big" John Mason for his client centred approach, support, and unique sense of humour. Both very close friends of many years, and, more importantly, they were there when I needed them. My thanks also must go to all the primary schools in Redcar and Cleveland who participated in the "Huge Bag of Worries" pilot, in particular Kevin Skelton from Ravensworth Junior School, who first spotted the potential of the "Huge Bag of Worries" and said yes!

Sticks and Stones

CONTENTS

Chapter 1   - A Northern Childhood

Chapter 2   - Angels with Dirty Faces

Chapter 3   - My Father

Chapter 4   - A New Direction

Chapter 5   - Understanding and Acceptance

Chapter 6   - Looking Beyond the Label

Chapter 7   - A Learning Experience

Chapter 8   - Victorian Values

Chapter 9   - The Wind of Change

Chapter10   - Pastures New

Chapter 11   - Returning to England

Chapter 12   - A Dark Place

Chapter 13   - A New Campaign

Chapter 14   - The Huge Bag of Worries

Chapter 15   - The Wider Community

Sticks and Stones

Chapter 16   - The Future

Appendices   - Articles Published by the Press

Sticks and Stones

Chapter 1 – A Northern Childhood

My childhood was unremarkable in many ways and on reflection not dissimilar to that of many other working class children growing up in the industrial North East of England during the 1960's and 1970's. I am the youngest of three children, with an older brother and sister. My birthplace, Staithes, is a small fishing village nestling beneath high cliffs looking out to the North Sea. Staithes is synonymous with one man, Captain James Cook, who lived and worked in the village before setting sail to discover Australia. It becomes a tourist haunt for many during the summer months, either to sunbathe on the beach, or to ramble along some of the scenic walks in the area such as the Cleveland Way.

As a family we were not poor as such, but neither were we rich. Our small coal fired terraced house was sandwiched between similar houses on a large council estate. It has changed little from the time when I grew up there all those years ago. All the houses were coal fired heated with no central heating. During dark winter evenings nobody would be able to distinguish the village from a distance as the smoke emitted from each chimney would blanket it in smog.

There was a strong sense of community growing up in the village. Everybody knew everybody else and help was always at hand if needed in a crisis.

Sticks and Stones

In many other parts of England I believe this community spirit has now gone. Doors are no longer left unlocked and crime is on the increase. People are not as trusting as then and who can blame them. We lived at the upper part of the village which is separated by a very steep bank. Most of the upper property was council owned and the lower part privately owned.

The lower part overlooks the sea and consists of many small cottages all huddled together. It is the lower part all the visitors flock to each year to visit with its picture postcard scenery and history. A small beck runs through the village where I spent many days of my childhood throwing sticks and stones into the water and searching for eels. The beck is overlooked by many dilapidated pigeon lofts and allotments, all synonymous with the culture and heritage of this part of the country.

Childhood was relatively uneventful until I reached the age of seven when I was to dice with death in an unexpected way. I was hit by a car whilst playing on our local green one dark December night. One minute I was excitedly running away from a friend who was chasing me, and the next I was lying in a crumpled heap on the side of the road.

Covered in blood, and in shock, I wondered what had happened. I remember at that moment trying to make sense of it all. Following the impact I found myself lying at the rear of the car

Sticks and Stones

surrounded by neighbours all wanting to help in whatever way they could. My friends stood around bewildered, all crying and wondering what had happened, wondering if it was somehow their fault. By chasing me had they forced me into the oncoming car?

Somebody brought me a blanket to protect me from the winter chill and hypothermia. It all seemed so unreal. I remember others all gazing at me from their doorsteps, all looking concerned. I waited for what seemed like an eternity for the ambulance to arrive. I lay covered in blood and my skin was punctured by dislodged pieces of grit, the result of being dragged along the road.

My left hand was torn to shreds, though I felt no pain. I was in a state of shock. If anything I was embarrassed by all the attention and feared being reprimanded by my parents for all the fuss I was causing and not following the green cross code.

My recently bought jeans were covered in blood and dirt and I recall feeling so guilty for soiling them. Blood was oozing from a puncture hole under my chin caused by a sharp jutting edge of the exhaust pipe. For a short distance the exhaust pipe had dragged me, like a rag doll, helpless along the road.

I had a profound fear of needles. As a precondition that I would go in the ambulance to hospital I sought reassurance from my mother that

Sticks and Stones

I wouldn't have to have any injections when I got there. This put her in a difficult position of course. She assured me that I wouldn't. Unfortunately she was somewhat economical with the truth. The last I saw of her that night was when she collapsed onto the roadside overcome by all the trauma. The first thing they did when I arrived at the hospital was cut away all my clothing and give me numerous injections.

As I was being stretchered into the ambulance I remember looking over at all the shocked faces watching from the front doorsteps of the houses, or peering through gaps in the curtains. The whole estate seemed to be watching my every move, no doubt all worrying what would become of the little lad from number 26, just round the corner.

This was a near fatal accident and I spent 3 months over the winter period, including Christmas, in hospital recovering and having surgery on my injuries.

As a consequence of the accident various parts of my body were left heavily scarred, mainly my left hand and shoulder, and under my chin.   I became emotionally traumatised and psychologically damaged for quite a while afterwards. This wasn't helped by the repeated playing on the ward of "Two Little Boys" by Rolf Harris which was the number one record at the time!

Whenever I hear that record the memories always

Sticks and Stones

come flooding back. My accident was a hugely significant event in my life that was to affect me for many years to come.

I would have regular vivid nightmares about the accident, reliving it in my dreams. The car was replaced by a large tiger chasing me for some unknown reason. I still cannot fathom that one out, but I am sure a Child Psychologist could, given the opportunity of getting me on the therapist's couch.

I experienced post traumatic stress disorder. My left hand became horribly disfigured from extensive skin grafting due to the excessive tissue damage. I felt ashamed about showing my scars to anybody, particularly my hand which was the most visible and unsightly. I wasn't a particularly confident child and this confidence level was further damaged. I felt like some kind of circus freak. Such was the extent of my scarring and my own exaggerated perception of this. My paranoia and over-sensitivity went into overdrive.

On the day I was to have the bandages removed from my hand and see the extent of the skin graft, and the resulting scars, I froze on the spot. The nurse stood at my side with a mirror. I sat on a wooden chair. Every time I moved my face to avoid looking at my disfigurement the nurse would strategically angle the mirror to ensure I would see it sooner or later. We played this cruel game for a couple of minutes until finally I relented and looked at my hand. I cried uncontrollably and the nurse

Sticks and Stones

hugged me to comfort my pain. I have forgotten many memories from my childhood, but this one remains vivid to this day.

I became so obsessed about my hand that I would eat my school dinners with my left hand behind my back for fear of putting the other children off their dinners. I didn't want to alarm them. I was overly considerate about not wanting to hurt or offend others, even to my own detriment. It was acceptable for me to not eat my own dinner as long as I didn't put the others off theirs.

The flexion and strength of my left hand would never be the same again, and my mother was warned that I may eventually have to have my hand amputated. Only time would tell. Thankfully this didn't happen. The scars may be unsightly but I still have the use of my hand, albeit with limitations. It became known as my "gammy hand" thus taking on a character and identity of its own. So everyone, especially family would refer to my hand as the gammy hand. In winter when the cold was biting it would change colours, a bit like a chameleon. Part of my hand would be blue and other parts red. This would draw even more unwanted attention and make me feel even more self-conscious.

For years afterwards when someone momentarily glanced at my left hand I would then be asked the same question; "How did you burn your hand?". I then found myself reliving the experience of the

Sticks and Stones

accident by having to correct their assumption. The less sensitive people would look aghast and grimace upon seeing my hand. That reaction would lower my self confidence even more. The more sensitive would remark "It doesn't really look that bad". This never fooled anyone, least of all me.

Adults as well as children would respond like this. After a while I became used to it. It came with the territory. In time I came to accept my hand and all its deformity. I was once told as an adult that it gave me a sense of character, it was unique to me. You can say that again. I took that as a compliment.

I excelled at nothing as a child and just seemed to "fit in." Academically I was never at the top of the class but I did enough to get by. I enjoyed playing football but was rarely picked for the school team. On the one occasion I was selected for the school team I was so overawed by the whole occasion I seemed to freeze in the middle of the pitch. It was pouring with rain and I stood bedraggled wearing an oversized pair of shorts and shirt. I remember the shirts were a throwback to the 1950s and this was the early seventies.

My legs were so thin my mother jokingly referred to me as "sparrow legs" Sometimes sensitivity wasn't her strongest point, but that said it was all taken in fun as it was intended to be. Despite already having a complex about my left hand the

Sticks and Stones

jokes were often as biting and piercing as the North Easterly winds we had become accustomed to.

I was substituted early into the second half as I was at that point making no positive contribution to the game whatsoever. I still think that the Manager picked me out of pity as I recall harassing him for weeks beforehand to be selected! I would probably have faired better in goal but too much catching of the ball would make my left hand painful. I had many friends as a child and a good sense of humour, one which I exploited to keep friends and attract new ones also. I played the joker most of the time which always went down well with my peers. I haven't changed much, still very self-deprecating and playing the joker.

I did possess good communication skills and a keen sense of survival. I was fairly streetwise. I was caring, although somewhat over-sensitive, and in many ways as an adult I still am. Some of these attributes were invaluable, particularly the communication skills, when avoiding situations such as local gang warfare, or escaping the local bully. This was the industrial North East in the Seventies where no prisoners were ever taken alive.

During one local football game my friends and I were ambushed on the way back to the coach. One of my friends was being overpowered and found an iron bar. He used it to good effect to

Sticks and Stones

defend himself, for days later he had an air of confidence and invincibility about him. He strutted along telling everyone he met how he "filled in" the thug who was holding him on the floor. He even shaved his head to play the part. This was during the rise of the far right, the National Front, and shaven heads were associated with aggression at the time. All to the sound of Slade and the wearing of Doctor Marten boots. The North East in the seventies seemed such a depressing place to be at times.

Sticks and Stones

Chapter 2 - Angels with Dirty Faces

Growing up in a fishing village in North Yorkshire ensured plenty of adventures; climbing high cliffs, playing on the beach, and rambling through the nearby Yorkshire moors during long hot summer months. It was idyllic. Night time would be spent playing football on the local council owned playing field, or stealing apples and conkers from nearby trees. The apples would all be gathered up and stuffed down my jumper. As we all desperately ran home before getting caught many would spill onto the road. The ones I was fortunate to retain would be surreptitiously eaten in my bedroom. I can still taste them now.

We would form gangs and would fight each other using sticks and stones and whatever else we could lay our hands on. In time our weaponry became more sophisticated to include home made bows and arrows, and the occasional gun with pellets. These certainly hurt when you felt one pierce your back or more sensitive parts of your anatomy. These battles would be fought in the nearby woods where we would lay in wait ready to pounce on our opponents.

During one skirmish I found myself stood without my stick facing the enemy. With only feet separating us he stooped to pick up a stone off the ground. I stood on his hand but he quickly pulled it away. We eyeballed each other for a few seconds,

Sticks and Stones

which seemed like minutes. He did what I didn't think he would do. Without any mercy, or hesitation, he threw the stone straight at me smashing my nose.

I vividly remember running home crying with blood pouring from the wound. I still bear the small scar inflicted that day all those years ago. It is easily discernible now on what is not the smallest of noses. The irony of it all was that we became quite good friends after that. We both lived on the same estate. The next day in school the teacher asked me how I had hurt myself. I looked straight at the culprit when I replied that I had fallen. Respect and honour among villains, expected even in our little world.

I would visit my grandparents who are more commonly referred to here in the North East as nana and granddad, as they also lived in the village along with other relatives. My uncle Jim was something of a local legend who remained a bachelor all his life. He would walk under the cliffs at first light every morning looking for driftwood which he would collect and carry home to chop into sticks for the fire. He would also sell bags of sticks to other villagers and visitors during the summer months. His strength defied science and human possibilities and would have been comparable to that of an ant, such was his ability to lift far greater weight than his actual body size. He weighed about 9 stones and would often be seen carrying long beams of wood on his

Sticks and Stones

shoulders with his dog, Asta, by his side. Often he would find what I perceived to be hidden treasures such as footballs, toys or just crates that had fallen from ships, mainly from Russia if I recall.

I was intrigued by the foreign writing on the sides of crates and he would tell me stories about the different countries of origin.

Most of these stories were tall to say the least. His face was rugged having endured many years of long hard winters surviving the cold and arduous conditions. He rarely seemed to wash and had a cleaner who would come in and keep his house clean and tidy. His preference was for black clothes which he wore all the time, along with a cap. I don't think I can ever remember seeing him without a cap on his head. Such was his eccentricity that once when he was going to go on the annual trip to Scarborough, a seaside town about 20 miles away, he dressed as a Chicago gangster. Al Capone himself would have been impressed. He was wearing his usual black trousers and had exchanged his black woollen jumper for a black shirt and white tie. His final touch was the wearing of white plimsolls which had been recently polished. Stuffed into his jacket pocket were the obligatory Woodbine cigarettes, or coffin nails as he would call them!

I would sit and watch him for hours chop sticks inside his dark cellar and he would regale me with his exaggerated stories. Sometimes I would sit on

Sticks and Stones

his front doorstep which was in the heart of the
village and watch all the visitors and locals go by.
Every year the village would hold an event called
Lifeboat Day which has been running for hundreds
of years and is still popular today. People would
dress in costumes and fancy dress and there
would be a 'nightgown parade' through the village
on the evening before the main day. Hundreds
would turn out wearing nightclothes and carrying
torches or candles, they would then walk down a
traditional route and a prize would be given for the
best dressed.

On the day itself the lifeboat would be on display
alongside local lifeboats from nearby towns and
they would collectively re-enact a life saving
operation by rescuing someone from the sea. All
with the assistance of a helicopter hovering above.
There would be stalls, a tombola, and various
games all manned and organised by the villagers.
The day was usually rounded off with a disco.
This was the main traditional summer event.

During the dark winter months I would play football
with friends, and sometimes alone, outside my
house. The garden gates would provide the
permanent goals and the street lights provided
the floodlights. Every now and again the game
would have to be momentarily stopped whilst a car
drove past to avoid being hit. Clearly I still hadn't
learnt my lesson from previous close encounters
with moving vehicles.

Sticks and Stones

This was the early Seventies when the volume of traffic on the road was far less than now, particularly on our impoverished estate where cars were few at the time. A lady across the road would often come out to reprimand me for continually hitting the ball against her gate, or kicking it into her front garden. I would apologise profusely but also felt a bit aggrieved that she had so rudely disrupted my game. This never happened on match of the Day. This lady is now well into her Eighties and still lives in the same house. Her gate has long been changed, but the fence still looks the same and painted the same colour as all the other fences on the estate.

The same street lights remain for any aspiring young footballer. Whenever as an adult I went home to visit my family this same lady would wave over and remark how well I had done with my life since leaving school. I would smile back sheepishly, feeling guilty about the stress my nightly football activity must have caused her all those years ago.

Occasionally, we would all congregate behind the social club on Saturday nights and listen to the groups playing. Under dark northern skies, and with only the light from the fire exit door to guide us, we would rummage through the dustbins searching for used bingo cards. These we would pretend were wads of money. They were usually covered in cigarette ash and stank of stale beer. All the same, we would put them in our pockets

Sticks and Stones

and pretend that we were rich.

Occasionally a fight would break out at the end of the evening when too much cheap booze had been consumed and the local 'hard cases' would want to square up. We would stand and watch before it was broken up, usually by a woman, and we would all be sent home. These were our role models, the local hard men who let their fists do the talking. They were respected by us and some of us would try to emulate them. We would all pretend to revel in this bare knuckle pugilism under the dim light of the social club, but if truth be told we all felt scared. It was bravado. In reality I think we struggled to understand what all this tribal blood-letting was about.

Sometimes the defeated fighter would make eye contact with me and for a split second look embarrassed. His face, along with his pride, had taken a battering, and now his humiliation was there for all the watching children, and adults, to see. I would search for specks of blood on the concrete following the fight before I went home and excitedly told my parents. This was the world I grew up in and all I understood to be normal at that time.

On New Years Eve a friend and I would stand outside the club waiting for the revellers to appear. One by one they would all give us money once we had wished them happy New Year. The more intoxicated someone was, the richer the pickings.

Sticks and Stones

In our small minds they were fair game. Again we would duck the punches from the fights that would invariably break out as it was well worth the risk. We would then run home with our pockets filled with coins, and sometimes notes.

This became a yearly event. What surprised me the most was the lack of interest from our peers, who were obviously oblivious to our yearly collections. I wouldn't feel safe allowing my children to engage in this activity. Nowadays knives have replaced fists as the weapon of choice, and life seems to be of less value. A different era altogether now.

Sticks and Stones

Chapter 3 – My Father

My father worked at the local school which I
attended. His job was to keep the school heated
during the bitterly cold northern winters. He
regularly took me along to watch him shovelling
coal into the boiler on Sunday afternoons. I was
eager to learn about what he did to keep the
school heated. On Sunday evenings there wasn't
usually much to do, especially during the winter
months, so I used to see this as an adventure. It
was ideal bonding time with my father, whom I
was very close to.

A lady used to help him occasionally, she held the
school keys and used to let us in to the buildings.
This was her responsibility and she supervised my
father's work. Whenever my father wasn't there
she would question me intensely about where he
went when not at work, and his "illness." I was
aware that he suffered with his "nerves" and
occasionally went into hospital for treatment for
this. This is what she was referring to. It was
common knowledge in the village that my father
experienced mental health problems, which were
referred to as "bad nerves."

Her questioning at times became a barrage of
questions, but there was no empathy or
compassion to these. I can clearly recall her
continual probing to find out more about my father,
and the problem he had with his "nerves". As a

Sticks and Stones

young boy I felt myself becoming embarrassed as a consequence of this ladies behaviour. I wondered why my father was so different to warrant all this attention.

Her interest seemed above and beyond anybody else's, It felt like emotional bullying. Whenever my father wasn't in the vicinity she would start probing me. I felt upset and angry and also ambivalent towards my father for seemingly being "different" from all my friends' fathers. I then felt guilty for having these thoughts. I felt sorry for him and it was at this point that I first came to understand the stigma that surrounds someone having a mental illness. If he had a physical illness her questioning and attitude wouldn't have been so upsetting to me. This is certainly how I felt at the time. A broken arm or a broken leg wouldn't have attracted the same interest this woman had when questioning me.

My father had his problems and as a consequence would often have to spend time in hospital having treatment. During the times when he was "away" very little was said. His illness wasn't really explained to us, such I feel was the stigma at the time. Our family got on with life as we always try to do here in the north east, we are survivors and at the end of the day we coped. We had no option. There were times when he wasn't hospitalised, and I still have happy memories of going to the football games, watching Middlesbrough Football club, or just going on

Sticks and Stones

holiday to Scarborough, or the local funfair in Redcar. At times I would just play fight with him at home, usual father and son stuff.

At Christmas my parents always made an effort to make the event as enjoyable as possible. They saved as much as they could to ensure we had lots of presents despite not having much money. I would sit in front of our open coal fire and wish the day could last forever. An effort was made by both parents to appear unified and I am grateful for that. The same Christmas day routine we had every year would be replicated with my own children, such were the happy memories I retained from childhood.

When I reached fourteen my life and world was to change when my parents separated and my father left home. I saw it coming but as with most children I was in denial. Fighting back tears, I waved at him as he walked down the path with a small suitcase in his hand. That was nearly 40 years ago and I haven't seen him since. The night before he left I helped him to pack his small case as he told me he was going to start a new life. I felt excited for him, such was my childhood innocence. Naively I assumed he would keep in touch and come back every now and again to see me, after all he may have fallen out with my mum but that didn't stop him loving me. I was wrong to assume. I did miss him for quite a while afterwards, but in time my feelings for him waned. We suppress our feelings to the back of our

Sticks and Stones

minds, this is often how we cope with such a thing as a loss. Although my father didn't die it felt like a death to me. It was the death of our relationship. My coping mechanism was to completely block him from my life and act as if he didn't exist. I have done that for all these years. It was easier that way and less painful.

After all these years I have convinced myself that his illness played a significant part in the circumstances of his departure, and his failure to keep in contact. By believing this I do not feel I have been personally rejected or disowned; the illness has made him behave in this way and for that reason I can empathise. It helps me to think in this way and brings a degree of resolution to the whole story.

Sticks and Stones

Chapter 4 – A New Direction

Early teenage years came and went in a rather mundane, uneventful way. I started drinking in the local pubs from the age of 16, though kept myself out of trouble. I lost contact with many school friends; some had chosen to be members of gangs and others had started working. We all went our separate ways. As for gangs, I wasn't interested in any of that sort of thing. As with most teenagers, I dated a few girls, though nothing serious developed in any relationship. However one girl who I met whilst she was on holiday in the village I did like very much, and I professed my undying love when she returned to Middlesbrough, her home town. It wasn't reciprocated. We exchanged a few letters written on regulation school writing paper but it fizzled out; holiday romances never seem to work anyway and we were both quite immature, especially me.

I got my first full time job working in a local scampi factory when I was 17. I worked on the processing section, it was hard graft standing on my feet all day in a smelly cold and wet environment. My left hand was badly affected by the continuous peeling of the shells, which were very hard. The skin tissue was much thinner following the accident and skin grafting, and my left thumb suffered the strain. I didn't have the same strength or flexion in my left thumb. I wore gloves but this made little or no difference. The

Sticks and Stones

scampi would then be breaded before it left the factory. I lasted about 6 months, and had to leave because of the damage to my hand.

At the age of eighteen I was desperate to leave the village and explore what life was like in other parts of the country. The job prospects were few in the area, and these were mainly in the fishing or mining industry. I never aspired to be a miner or a fisherman. I wasn't brave enough to venture down a mine, and I don't have a love of water so if I was to find work that would appeal to me I had to leave the area. I wanted to escape village life. I was starting to feel claustrophobic. I felt the urge to explore the world, or at least somewhere different.

I left home to go and stay with my cousins in Witham in Essex to try my luck there. I got a job in a local hotel as a waiter. Waiting and I were not really compatible and after about 3 months I left. I possessed a very broad north eastern accent and a certain naivety and immaturity that I wasn't proud of. I don't think this was very much appreciated or understood in a 4 star middle class rural Essex restaurant, where the clientele were mainly businessmen and women who expected service to be of the highest standard.
Compassion and patience wasn't their strongest points. I wasn't the most careful and coordinated of waiters and spilt the occasional soup and gravy which didn't go down too well among the guests. I couldn't blame my left hand for this though, I was just clumsy. My dialect also meant that certain

Sticks and Stones

words and sentences were completely altered and misinterpreted, often in an unintentionally humorous way. My pronunciation of "avocado" became "have a car door" which caused some consternation to say the least! I could see the funny side but those who took themselves too seriously couldn't.

One day after a very busy morning and lunch routine the manager took me into his office and told me I had to improve or I would be dismissed, or words to that effect. I felt quite hurt as I had always turned up for duty, sometimes at 5.30 in the morning for the breakfast shift, which very few other staff were keen on working. I believed I had tried my best and it wasn't easy being so young and so far away from home. That was my excuse anyway, but this didn't seem to cut any ice with him, unfortunately. I left his office and returned to the kitchen to a mountain of glasses that needed to be washed from the previous evening. I picked up a glass and thought "I've had enough of this", I then grabbed my coat from the hanger and walked out without another word being spoken. I never went back and then returned north with my self esteem dented somewhat, but at least I had learnt how to fold a napkin, a skill which I have remembered to this day but don't often have to put into practice!

I was now back in the North East and thinking about what to do next. I still didn't have any clear plans as far as a career went, but wanted to work

Sticks and Stones

as I didn't like being on the dole; my friends were all in work and I needed the stimulation and interest work offered, as well as a regular wage. One day whilst doing my usual search of the jobs page in our local newspaper I came across an advertisement for a hospital porter's job. It was in a psychiatric hospital just outside London. This interested me. I thought that this would be a good opportunity for me to travel again to another area, make new friends, and experience what life was like behind the walls of a psychiatric hospital. I only knew what I had seen on the television and read in the newspapers, and of course this was often sensationalised and distorted, so I could see for myself how true this really was.

I also thought that I may at the same time meet others who experience mental illness and thereby understand more about the condition that my father suffered from. Little did I appreciate at the time that I would eventually go on to train to be a mental health nurse, and spend the next 27 years working within psychiatric nursing. Or that I would later dedicate my life to challenging the stigma my father faced, and many like him experience daily.

In March 1979 as snow blanketed the North East of England I headed south on the train to Fairfield Hospital in Hertfordshire. I carried a small battered suitcase, not dissimilar to the one my father had left home with, that had clearly seen better days holding inside all my worldly belongings. These didn't amount to very much. I

Sticks and Stones

felt a sense of adventure not knowing what awaited me. The hospital was situated between the towns of Stotfold and Letchworth, and set in over 200 acres of beautiful countryside. Fairfield could be described as a typical asylum type hospital being geographically isolated in keeping with the Victorian attitude of socially ostracising the mentally ill. Between 1860 and 1898 it had been called the Three Counties Asylum, it now had the more modern and respectable title of Fairfield Hospital.

As I wandered through the endless shiny corridors I was taken aback by the sheer size and beauty of the place. It was all very beguiling. The inside resembled all the old films I recalled as a child which depicted asylums, and it was so stereotypical of those. In fact it felt as if I had stepped back in time onto a film set. There was a sense of unreality to it all. A gothic facade with an imposing tower set the scene, with high ceilings, ornate brickwork, and long shiny polished corridors stretching as far as the eye could see. It was hauntingly beautiful. Staff and patients paced the corridors night and day and It housed over 1,000 patients and a similar number of staff.

Fairfield was a thriving community, and as large as any small town. The hospital had a quintessential English feel. It was surrounded by trees, winding lanes and the obligatory church. It had a bowling green and a cricket and football pitch. This was rural Hertfordshire, not as stunning or rugged as

Sticks and Stones

the Yorkshire I had left behind, but beautiful all the same.

I quickly settled into my job as a porter and started to familiarise myself with my new surroundings. I still possessed a very broad northern accent so endured the usual teasing about being a northerner, and having a penchant for pigeons, whippets, and cloth caps. It goes with the territory. In reality I had none of these, but I went along with the banter and made the effort to make new acquaintances. I knew I had to learn to be somewhat thick skinned. I enjoyed the spirit of community at the hospital. I still miss that now.

I was placed in accommodation that had clearly seen better days. It was a second world war barracks building, housing myself and other domiciliary staff. The Ritz it certainly wasn't. I had a very small room in which one would have had difficulty swinging a kitten, never mind a cat. We all shared a communal shower with primitive washing facilities and toilets. It was called Hut 4, the name itself conjuring up visions of a concentration camp. It was centrally heated and had a lounge and a small kitchen which was rarely used. Most of the food we would get from the hospital canteen or local takeaways.

I began making friends and started getting used to the banter and camaraderie. We were all men sharing all male accommodation. Many jokes were played, especially on the new arrivals at the

Sticks and Stones

hospital sharing accommodation in notorious Hut 4. One of the first people I met, and became very close friends with, was Webby, a Geordie porter colleague. His name was John Webb, and he had the nickname of Webby. Webby had a sense of humour second to none and was always playing tricks on people. One night we were all sitting watching TV and were very hungry. The canteen was closed and very few of us ever bothered to shop and cook our own meals. Webby asked if any of us wanted fish and chips from the local take away in the village. He said he would go down on his push-bike to collect them as it was a 20 minute walk and we were all weary from a hard days work. We jumped at the chance, all grateful for his generosity, and thoughtfulness.

As the cliché goes we should have smelt a rat, but we didn't. 20 minutes later Webby returned holding a bundle of newspaper in his hands and urging someone to get the plates as it was very hot. I grabbed a plate and stood waiting for him to unwrap the fish and chips. He unwrapped his bundle of newspaper and to my shock a hedgehog dropped onto my plate. I don't know who was the most shocked, the hedgehog or me. I didn't know whether to laugh or cry. He remains a good friend now 30 years later and his sense of humour remains as unpredictable and unorthodox now as it was then. The hedgehog was safely placed back outside in the bushes, somewhat perplexed at what had happened.

Sticks and Stones

The hospital became a thriving, bustling place during the day with everybody going about their different businesses. Within the main building were a number of shops, and a large Recreational Hall where at Christmas the pantomime would run for staff and patients. There was a WRVS canteen where people would pop in for a coffee and to socialise. And of course there was the essential watering hole, the staff social club. Many people met future wives or husbands within its basic facilities, and it was within these basic confines that I met my wife Teresa a year after starting at the hospital. Our eyes were to meet across a cigarette ash and beer stained table at the Saturday night disco. Everyone from the hospital and the surrounding villages seemed to go to the Saturday night disco. What I think is quite ironic is the amount of trouble that would take place there.

The club stood in the centre of a very large hospital and almost on a weekly basis a fight or two, or three, would break out. Now we are all led to believe that the most dangerous people are incarcerated in a secure ward in a psychiatric hospital. Or in prison!

Dangerous people who were not deemed to be suffering from a mental illness caused mayhem at this disco, and the regular doorman had his work cut out controlling them all. I find this somewhat ironic. In hindsight most of the weekly revellers would have felt safer being on the wards where glasses and punches were seldom thrown.

Sticks and Stones

A large cricket and football pitch adjoined the social club, with a small bowling green tucked in between. All were surrounded by an assortment of trees and bushes. Most of the wards were based within the beautiful main building, but it also had a number of wooden barrack style accommodation blocks dating back to the second World War. These housed the elderly patients, or geriatrics as they used to be referred to. Surprisingly enough this area was referred to as the hutted area.

Most of the hospital's 200 acres or so of land was made up of fields and greenery of one type or another. During the warm summer months it became one of the most tranquil and scenic places anyone could visit to wile away the time. The locals appreciated the grounds because of their beauty and would often walk their dogs or just stroll through them. On the periphery of the grounds were the blue and green lagoons, two romantically named quarry sites that were also places to escape for solitude. These were idyllic surroundings that I took advantage of as much as possible during the warm weather.

I had been at the hospital for about 6 months and now had a routine around work and play, mostly play. This consisted of drinking, chatting up the female nurses with little success most of the time, shopping, and going to rock concerts. These were usually at the Hammersmith Odeon, or the

Sticks and Stones

Rainbow theatre in London. Shortly before Christmas 1979 I was looking forward to going to see Queen with a couple of my porter colleagues at the Rainbow theatre. I arranged to meet a friend for lunch on the day. We met at a well known fast food outlet in Hitchin town centre. It was bustling with people all out to do their Christmas shopping as it was market day, and there was an air of excitement around the place. This was to change in a most dramatic and murderous way.

As we sat eating our meals our attention was drawn to a couple standing near the entrance who were arguing. As with most other people we tried to ignore this and continued with our conversation, though the arguing became more intense and it was becoming more difficult to ignore. Suddenly I heard a scream and someone shout "she's been stabbed". The woman was a large West Indian lady who was wearing a very thick fur coat, the man she was arguing with was also West Indian and when I looked over again he had run off . He had stabbed her. Both my friend and I jumped up and walked to where the lady was now slumped on the floor being cradled by another elderly white lady. The lady was reassuring her that everything will be OK but we watched as she took her last breath and died in front of us all. She was surrounded by her many shopping bags which no doubt held Christmas presents. I was shocked and couldn't believe what I had witnessed, all within a matter of minutes, life and then death.

Sticks and Stones

The ambulance arrived shortly after but it was now too late. Everyone started to leave the restaurant and go their different ways, all equally shocked at what they had witnessed. Little was said by anyone. I looked down at the floor where the lady had been stabbed and saw a small patch of blood, so small it could easily have been missed, it was barely noticeable. The lady's heavy fur coat must have absorbed the blood loss resulting from her stab wounds. I later found out she had been stabbed a couple of times by her estranged husband, he had then run off down a nearby alleyway, only to be arrested later that evening in a pub, drinking.

I made my way back to my accommodation on the bus and couldn't stop thinking about what had happened. I began questioning myself as to if I could have done anything to stop this murder, it had all happened within minutes and didn't appear to have been a premeditated act of violence. One minute they were talking, the next minute they were arguing, and the next minute she was dead. When I got off the bus I went straight to the staff social club and ordered a pint of beer to calm my nerves. The barmaid asked if I had seen a ghost because I was as white as a sheet and still in shock as I explained the incident I had just witnessed. I went to the concert that night but my thoughts kept drifting to that poor woman and her shopping bags. Her dying face is something I will always remember alongside the compassion of the old lady who held her as she passed away.

Sticks and Stones

Chapter 5 – Understanding and Acceptance

On visiting the many wards I would befriend the patients and they would tell me all about the problems that led to their admissions. A large number of the patients had been in hospital for many years, and many lacked the daily living skills to cope back in the community, the "outside world". They had become institutionalised. They had come to regard the hospital as their home and as such felt safe and secure within the hospital walls. Many of the patients had marked social skills deficits, this being the devastating symptoms of the illnesses they had, such as schizophrenia. However, they didn't match the negative stereotype I and many others had of so-called "mental patients". My own perceptions and preconceived ideas were shattered when meeting these people. They exhibited some bizarre behaviour as a consequence of their illnesses, but this did not frighten me. In fact the opposite was the case. Many had a certain character and warmth that was endearing. They were trusting of those who were there to care for them and this made them feel secure.

One gentleman, George, whom I got to know well, had a remarkably traumatic history. George had been a teacher in Germany during the second world war. The Nazis were on the rise and for anyone unsympathetic to their cause Germany was a dangerous place to live and work. George

Sticks and Stones

was ordered to hang a picture of Hitler on the classroom wall. He bravely refused. He showed incredible courage and conviction by taking this stance. As a consequence of his insubordination George found himself hauled into prison and tortured for showing disrespect to the fuehrer. His life was to change irreversibly.

As a consequence of his torture and maltreatment at the hands of his captors George became severely mentally ill. He would never teach again. His spirit was broken, his mind was in pieces. George required intense hospitalisation on his return to England. I got to know George well. By this time he was shabbily dressed and extremely institutionalised. Though old, he still walked with a spring in his step.

His days would be spent wandering aimlessly from one part of the hospital to another, sometimes muttering incoherently to those who chose to listen. He still retained a powerful intellect, though he was easily angered and suffered fools badly. One day he would say hello and the next he would respond with an insult. Sometimes he would do both in the same breath. It seemed to be all around timing and catching him on a good day.

Occasionally George would converse with me about cricket, a sport which he was passionate about, and politics. He had a deep loathing for Margaret Thatcher, who was the premier at the time. The mention of her name would be enough

Sticks and Stones

to stir anger and disdain. George's views were very left wing and from what I can recall he regarded himself as a staunch Marxist. At times when engaging George in conversation, looking into his eyes I could see they were lifeless, the light had long been snuffed out. Such was the torment he still endured.

One wet and miserable night I was walking from one area of the hospital to return to my living quarters. I heard George's easily recognisable voice call from the bushes. What he was doing in the bushes I can only guess. The rain was now lashing down and we both stood talking under the dimly lit street light. George wanted to inform me of his opinion of Margaret Thatcher, no change there then. I just wanted to escape the downpour and dry out. His clothes were becoming saturated but this did not deter George, he had a story to tell and I was the one he had chosen to listen. I eventually persuaded George to go inside as we were both at risk of hypothermia at this point, or drowning, or both!

As I reminisce I wonder how anyone can abuse or belittle George because of his eccentricity or differences. It wasn't appropriate to stand and talk in the middle of a monsoon on a cold winter night, but to George this was acceptable because I chose to stand and listen. His voice had been silenced all those years previously but not now. I was someone who was prepared to listen and converse. George wasn't going to let that

Sticks and Stones

opportunity slip away and I don't blame him.

To an outsider ignorant of his past and his illness George may have been perceived as a tramp, a nobody, someone who lacked personal hygiene and self respect through laziness. Others like myself who were very fond of George knew differently. We admired his bravery and tenacity against all the odds. Here we saw someone who was inspirational to ourselves. The fact that he was mentally ill was of no significance, why should this have a bearing on his character? Torture and abuse by others meant George was destined to spend the rest of his days incarcerated within an institution, living in his own world and completely institutionalised. And this was no dream world. His world was not a nice place to be, it was a dark and lonely place and one that held many secrets that George would have taken to his grave.

George was just one example. I recall having many misconceptions challenged and destroyed upon meeting the long stay patients. Some with their idiosyncratic, eccentric ways, having picked up learnt behaviour, the result of spending many years in an institution.

Sticks and Stones

Chapter 6 – Looking Beyond the Label

I soon realised when meeting the patients and engaging in conversation with them that it was so important to look beyond the label of the illnesses, such as schizophrenia, or manic depression, now termed bipolar affective disorder, and see the unique individual on the other side. A person's character should not be defined by their illness, and sadly in the case of the mentally ill this is all too often the case. This was one of the first lessons I learnt when arriving at the hospital and meeting the patients for the first time.

I struck up a friendship with a young lady, Anne, who was an inpatient on one of the female wards. All the wards were single sex. In time nationally they would become mixed, and now it has returned to single sex wards again. Anne would joke and exchange banter with myself and my porter colleagues. She was the same age as us, nineteen, and barely an adult. I would stand holding my mop in the corridor and Anne would tease me for having acne and being so quiet, all typical teenage banter. On one of my visits to the ward I noticed she wasn't there, which was unusual as she always greeted me knowing I would deliver the meals at around the same time daily. When I enquired as to where she was I was informed by a member of staff that she had seriously harmed herself during the night and was receiving treatment in the local General Hospital.

Sticks and Stones

In many ways this was a reality check for me, and brought home the realisation that I was in a psychiatric hospital. It was the nature of the beast, these incidents went with the territory I was told at the time. I remember at that moment taking stock of my life and appreciating how lucky I was in comparison. I had friends, a job, accommodation and a carefree attitude to life. An immaturity yes, but more importantly I had good self esteem which Anne clearly didn't have.

We had laughed and joked the day before and I was oblivious to her suffering. It was well hidden, it was masked perfectly. It seemed like we had much in common, but in reality we were like chalk and cheese. I had experienced a fairly happy, contented childhood, albeit with certain events causing trauma along the way. Anne wasn't as fortunate.

As a child she had endured abuse from her father both physically and emotionally, thus resulting in her having such self loathing as to want to kill herself. And all this at the tender age of nineteen. Anne survived and in time returned to the hospital bearing the emotional and physical scars of her ordeal. I for one was pleased and reassured to see her again.

Having worked as a porter for two years I was approached one day by a Senior Nursing Officer who asked if I had ever considered nursing as a career. It had been brought to her attention that I

Sticks and Stones

had been observed talking to the patients in the corridor and on the wards, and news spread quickly within the hospital. She commented about my friendly nature and I appreciated this. A career in caring was something she was encouraging me to think seriously about. I was extremely flattered by her interest and following her suggestion applied for a job as a nursing assistant. I was now twenty years of age.

Many years have passed since this lady encouraged me to go into nursing and our paths haven't crossed since. I am eternally grateful for having been given the encouragement at the time. It was to change the whole course of my life. I would like to think after all these years that I haven't let her down. That is for others to judge.

I was successful in the interview and found myself working on the wards as a Nursing Assistant. It was both exciting and also daunting as I appreciated the new-found responsibility I had now acquired. I already knew many of the staff and patients which was an advantage. I was also familiar with the geographical layout of all the wards and grounds, and to some degree the different daily routines on the wards.

On meeting many of the patients on the wards I began to learn in more depth about the different conditions they suffered from. In time this understanding and newly acquired knowledge would help me to understand more about my

Sticks and Stones

father's illness. I came to appreciate that many people struggled with their illnesses in similar ways to himself. His condition wasn't unique.

As a child I had always looked upon my father's illness with the same stigma and embarrassment that others had. Consequently I am embarrassed now all these years later because of that. However, I was only a child influenced by all the adults around me. Those elders who I was meant to look upon as role models and respect. This is my defence. To some degree I could be forgiven for this. What was their excuse?

The lady who insisted on asking personal questions impervious to my discomfort. Similarly others who may make derogatory remarks when gossiping, some of whom I would imagine would have held negative views about mental illness. Staithes was no different to any other small village or town at the time where ignorance and misunderstanding surrounding mental illness existed. It goes on now in every town and village in the country.

Many of the patients I met were clearly very ill, and as such required long term treatment within a hospital environment. As a consequence of their illnesses and hospitalisation their families also experienced the loss I had felt as a child. Whenever someone experiences a mental breakdown it isn't only the patient who suffers, it is also the family and loved ones. Often they are left

Sticks and Stones

to pick up the pieces at home, alone, and are expected to cope with the gossip and the rumours. The family unit is broken, as mine was all those years ago.

I now found myself having more dedicated time as part of my daily duties to engage more with each patient, and in doing so learnt about their conditions and treatment plans. I felt privileged that people were willing to trust me and open up to disclose personal information to me. I had to earn the respect of each and every patient and didn't expect to be shown it just because I wore a nurse's uniform.

I was determined to show the Nursing Officer I had what it took to be a good nurse. These qualities are many, such as compassion, empathy, a non judgemental attitude, and genuineness. All these qualities are pivotal when counselling people and forging good therapeutic relationships. The Nursing Officer had placed her trust in me by encouraging me to go into nursing. I wasn't for letting her down and was determined to prove myself.

Sticks and Stones

Chapter 7 – A Learning Experience

The first ward I found myself working on was a Continuing Care ward which had around 20 patients, mostly with a diagnosis of schizophrenia. The patients had been in hospital for many years and realistically most were expected to spend their remaining days there, such was the severity of their illnesses, and institutionalised behaviour. In many ways this was a relatively easy kind of ward to start working on, as opposed to the more stressful secure or acute admission wards. I found this work very enjoyable and soon became familiar with the daily routine and each patient's idiosyncratic ways. During the day most of the patients would attend one of the therapy departments, stay on the ward, or just wander around the grounds of the hospital. The ward had a well used pool table and a cosy lounge with TV and radio. The ward décor was generic, all the wards, male and female, were painted the same NHS standard colours and lacked imagination and originality. There wasn't much of a homely individual feel differentiating one ward from another. One of the patients, Ronald, was an excellent pool player and I would spend many hours wiling the time away playing pool with him. It would be accurate to say that Ronald was tortured by the voices he heard almost constantly and had a diagnosis of paranoid schizophrenia. He would have persecutory delusional thoughts and was always shouting in response to the

Sticks and Stones

voices he heard, sometimes they would never
ease up and his face was often pained due to the
constant insulting remarks.

In the middle of a game he would stop and shout
in response to his accuser, and then apologise to
me for his distraction. If a female was in the
vicinity Ronald would apologise profusely for his
language. He was a gentleman who had been
brought up in an era where swearing in front of
ladies was unforgivable; it just wasn't acceptable.
I would try to reassure him and distract him hoping
that this would bring some relief, but it rarely
worked. To an outsider this would have looked
strange and somewhat comical, the sight of
Ronald occasionally shouting at nothing and me
standing observing, though comical it definitely
wasn't. It would have been difficult for the most
hardened of men to not feel compassion and
sympathy for Ronald. He was totally trapped in a
world where he was constantly persecuted by his
own mind. Medication did little to ease his torture
and sleep would have been the only time he ever
had any respite.

After about a year I found myself transferred to the
locked male secure ward. Here I found myself
working with more challenging patients in a
constantly locked, secure environment. In the late
1970's the padded cell was still in use, this being a
throwback to the days of custodial care. The male
secure ward was the only ward which housed the
padded cell. This room would be used only as a

last resort, as it was intended to be. All other alternatives such as medication and de-escalating techniques such as talking, persuasion and reassurance were to be considered first, before the room became the only way of containing a dangerous situation.

The safety of the other patients and staff had to be taken into consideration whenever someone became violent and beyond reason. I didn't like the use of the padded cell at all. It blew in the face of all that I had come into nursing for. Whenever I found myself involved in a restraining situation, and the room became an inevitable conclusion, I viewed this as the only option open to ensure everyone's safety. This included the patient being restrained. In the absence of effective medication/ treatment at the time there was little alternative. It was something that as nurses we had to work with, but I would like to think the majority of nurses I worked with always viewed this as the last option to consider, the restriction of someone's freedom and movement.

The secure ward housed patients who were generally deemed to be a danger to the public, and sometimes themselves, but required secure hospital ward based treatment as opposed to prison incarceration. This was usually determined by the courts when sentencing. The patients were mainly suffering from aggressive personality disorders or paranoid schizophrenia. The staff on the wards were nurses and not prison officers and as such the care given was to be therapeutic. Nurses not jailers - it was important to make that distinction. Many of the patients had offended through a lack of insight into their conditions and often not receiving the necessary treatment, rather than just being 'criminals'.

Occasionally I would be sent to other wards if they were short staffed due to sickness or holidays, but most of the time I would work on the secure ward. The other wards that I would find myself sent to were mostly caring for the elderly, then termed geriatric wards. On the secure ward I would assist the qualified staff in distributing medication, observation, and engaging in therapeutic activities on and off the ward, such as the therapy units. The ward also had a pool table and table tennis table which were well used.

The early 1990's heralded the removal of the archaic padded cells on all wards and the introduction of more humane seclusion rooms. It wasn't a day too soon and nobody mourned their passing. I certainly didn't. The padded cell did nothing to change people's perceptions of mental illness, and how the mentally ill were treated. It only served to perpetuate the stigma and misunderstanding around treatment programmes in society.

At the time medication wasn't as effective as it is now, and often the patient would be left to experience extreme side effects such as

Sticks and Stones

excessive salivation, a shuffling gait, and mannerisms that drew unwanted attention to them. Often the side effects perpetuated the stigmatizing process all the more. Some patients even remarked to me that the side effects from the medication were often worse than the illness itself. I fully empathised with them.

Having worked as a Nursing Assistant for two years I had gained valuable experience on specialised wards treating a variety of conditions. I enjoyed the work immensely and made many new friends in the process. My wife Teresa had now qualified and encouraged me to seriously think about doing my Mental Health Nurse training. I applied to the School of Nursing and sat the required entrance test and passed. It was April 1982. As the Falklands War raged I found myself donning a student's tunic and attending the School of Nursing at the hospital. I could now put all the practical experience and knowledge that I had gained over the previous two years to good use. Certainly having spent those two years working as a Nursing Assistant prepared me well for the challenges ahead.

As a student I gained more knowledge and general awareness about the different medications used to treat the different psychiatric conditions. I became more involved in care planning and so many other aspects of nursing that as a nursing assistant I wouldn't have had as much involvement in. I had to also familiarise myself

Sticks and Stones

with the workings of legal legislation such as the Mental Health Act. My theoretical knowledge was increased significantly, and I also felt more confident about questioning practices on the wards. As a student I was actively encouraged to do this.

Some of the older staff, who had worked at the hospital for many years, often felt threatened when a student would start working on their wards and questioning their practices. Many staff were as institutionalised as many of the long stay patients, and reluctant to change. Old habits die hard.

I was though extremely fortunate to meet many staff who were exemplary in their delivery of a patient centred approach. I am indebted to those staff that went the extra mile to ensure the student experience was a positive one. I learnt a great deal from these staff, and I remember my tutor encouraging all of us to use the good staff on the wards as positive role models. I would endeavour to replicate their particular approaches and style of nursing.

Chapter 8 – Victorian Values

The hospital was old and many of the practices likewise and even anachronistic. Some were still Victorian. One example of an outdated policy on the wards was the colour coded cup system. All the cups on the wards were all colour coded. All the pink cups were for patient use only, and the green cups were for staff. I viewed this as being quite divisive and stigmatizing. I was surprised that nobody seemed to question this colour coded ruling.

My thoughts at the time were that we should be constantly reflecting on our own practices and whether these help or hinder the stigmatizing process. If we stigmatize the patients within the hospital by sharing negative views such as the particular colour code of cups and saucers, how can we successfully challenge the stigma outside of the hospital? We were in collusion with the bigots in society who hold the belief of locking people up and throwing away the key.

As my level of confidence grew I became more confident in using humour when talking to staff and patients. Humour is necessary when working within such a stressful role and is often very dark. Humour can be used to break down barriers and forge good relationships. It is also cathartic when used appropriately for the staff and the patient .

Sticks and Stones

In my approach to each and every patient I tried to
display a more personal side to me than being "a
nurse". I am not one dimensional. By this I mean
sharing some more personal information about
other aspects of my life, such as my hobbies and
interests, and my family. I am Lol the nurse, but I
am also Lol the father, and the husband, and the
friend. I would use this approach as I felt it helped
to break down barriers when meeting people and
being actively involved in their care plans, or
interventions as they are most commonly called.

Half way through my training and I was to spend 6
weeks gaining experience within a medical setting
of a general hospital. I was to spend this time at
Bedford General hospital. I enjoyed this
placement as it gave me an insight into the
workings of the general teams, and also an
awareness of the different conditions
compared with what I had been used to treating in
psychiatry. I was to witness those unfortunate to
suffer a heart attack and require de fibrillating, and
also have endoscopies and gastroscopies as part
of their treatment. The work was very much hands
on and task orientated and so far removed from
what I was accustomed to. There wasn't the time
to sit and talk to patients which I was used to
doing, I was emptying bedpans and helping to bed
bath patients. I learnt all about dressings and
ulcer care.

The staff all seemed to take me under their wings,
I was still in my early twenties and had much to

Sticks and Stones

learn. It was only a short placement and I wasn't expected to learn too much apart from a basic grasp of the workings of the team in a busy medical ward. It was a good experience for me. It gave me an insight into the demands and pressures of working on an acute busy medical ward.

Upon completing my training I now found myself fully qualified and raring to go! I was now in a stronger position to put many of my ideas into practice, having more autonomy now as a qualified nurse. That said, I still had much to learn from my mentors.

There is a saying in psychiatry that you only start to really learn once you have qualified and taken charge of a ward. In many ways this is true. You are still quite dependent on the older more experienced staff, and your own confidence level still has to grow with different experiences and situations that arise. The buck stops here.

We all learn from life experiences and nursing is no different, it is a continual learning process. It is always changing and evolving. This is in relation to all the different paperwork, research based practices being introduced, and particular incidents on the wards and whether these are managed effectively or not. At the moment mental health nursing is undergoing many great changes Nationally that hopefully will be for the betterment of the patients. Time will tell.

Sticks and Stones

I would feel a great sense of personal satisfaction when discharging someone who I had nursed for many weeks, sometimes months, with acute depression and they were now well enough to be discharged home. It was always a ward team effort, but I always felt pleased that I too had played a part in their recovery. After all these years that feeling hasn't waned.

I was to see many patients recover and go home to not be readmitted. Sadly I also saw patients discharged to either return again not long after, or more tragically commit suicide. Thankfully I can only count on one hand the number of patients I had nursed who had taken their lives over the past 27 years, but that is still too high a figure.

It is not easy to deal with when this happens because understandably, as a nurse, one always wonders whether more could have been done to prevent this. Those early years upon qualifying were enjoyable times but also testing times. It was a learning curve like no other. As well as being on my first ward when a patient committed suicide whilst on home leave, I also experienced the suicidal death of a colleague. I had regarded this person as a friend/ mentor as well as a colleague, and learnt a great deal from him when I first started working on the ward.

My colleague was dual trained as a General and also a Mental Health Nurse. He had a quiet,

Sticks and Stones

unassuming manner, and did his job in a professional way without too much fuss. Upon qualifying I looked for a positive role model and he exemplified what being a good nurse was all about. He was depressed but had masked this well. I was still relatively young and inexperienced and maybe had I been older he might have found confidence in confiding in me. This could have avoided the consequence of his suicide, who knows?

He had taken me under his wing, and imparted his extensive knowledge and experience to me, which I was grateful for. The thought did for quite a while ruminate in my head as to whether I could have done anything to prevent both deaths. I wrestled with my conscience and I do not think I could have done things differently as both were equally determined to end their suffering. Both patient and nurse were in their thirties, and this is what I regarded at the time as the futility of it all.

For the following two years I continued to work on the male admission unit and lived in a small flat with my partner, Teresa, within the hospital grounds and a stone's throw from the unit where I worked.

Chapter 9 – The Wind of Change

In January 1986 after being at the hospital for seven years it was time for a new challenge. I was now married to Teresa who is also a nurse. Hertfordshire was an expensive place in which to buy a house, and both of us yearned to return back "up north" to settle. There were no posts advertised at the nearest hospital to home in the North East, St Lukes in Middlesbrough, so we applied for posts at Whittingham Hospital near Preston in Lancashire.

Going to Whittingham was certainly an experience like never before, as the hospital had a reputation which we were blissfully unaware of when we applied. During the early 1970's a number of malpractices were alleged to have taken place there involving widespread abuse of patients. These were even discussed in the House of Lords, such was their severity and the concern they had caused.

I was informed of its awful history when I started working on the wards on permanent night duty, which was the post I had acquired. Basically, I was asked by one of the staff "why on earth did you come to work here?" Such was the continued reputation from all those years previously.

Whittingham was somewhat outdated in many

Sticks and Stones

ways, and its appearance was like something straight out of a gothic horror film. As with Fairfield it typified the old Victorian asylum. The hospital was socially isolated from Preston, the nearest large town, amidst hundred of acres of countryside near to the village of Goosnargh. Chingle Hall, which was once reputed to be the most haunted house in England, was also situated nearby. The scene was set.

Whittingham hospital at one point held the title of the largest asylum in Europe. I wouldn't have questioned that statistic. Whereas Fairfield had a population of over a thousand patients, Whittingham housed over three and a half thousand. This was in its "heyday". This number was around one thousand when I worked there. It was a huge complex of separate wards covering a very large area.

It was like stepping back in time again, and left me with the same feeling I had when I initially arrived at Fairfield. Whilst it didn't have the same regal elegance of Fairfield in its facade design and colour, Whittingham did have a daunting presence. It was certainly impressive, with an atmosphere second to none.

Whereas Fairfield was built from grey stone, and a listed building, Whittingham was built from the red brick, so synonymous with Lancashire. It lacked the aesthetic beauty and grace of Fairfield, but it was more structurally imposing.

Sticks and Stones

I was to work for two years on continuous night duty on mainly long stay wards, but also for a while on the acute admission unit. I made many friends both of staff and patients at the hospital, and it was disheartening that the hospital had such a negative reputation. Many staff were hard working, caring individuals. They had come into nursing like myself, with a desire to help others, and provide a high standard of individual care to each and every patient. A number of staff clearly somehow felt sullied because of events years previously and beyond their control. They bore the ghosts of the past, and the stigma that surrounded the hospital locally was more obvious than at Fairfield.

This wasn't aided of course by the fact that abuse was alleged to have taken place, and the reputation of the hospital had suffered irreparably as a consequence. The allegations of wet towels being used to abuse the patients at Whittingham only fuelled the long-standing myths of wet towel treatment being a norm within psychiatric establishments. I was also told by staff of bonfires being lit and case notes being burnt to hide the evidence of malpractice. Rumours and gossip were rife about its dreaded past.

Working on night duty over a long period is quite wearing and can be de-motivating. To some degree many staff feel de-skilled. They are not at the "cutting edge" of nursing because most of the time everybody sleeps. Their function is to ensure

Sticks and Stones

everybody has a comfortable nights rest. During the daytime there are Ward Rounds and numerous other activities, such as Occupational Therapy, to keep both staff and patients busy. There is also more time to sit and talk to the patients, and engage in recreational activities on the ward.

I was beginning to feel de-skilled working regular night duties so after two years thought very carefully about a fresh challenge, preferably on day duty, and in another area and another hospital. Both Teresa and I still yearned to return to my native North East to settle down. Whittingham at this point was facing closure as the late 1980's and early 1990's heralded the closure of many asylum type hospitals in favour of purpose built units. The old hospitals were now anachronistic. More modern residential and nursing homes were being built nationally to house those who needed care and accommodation. The Care in the Community Act launched in 1990 proposed this would go some way to promoting social inclusion. The aim of the act primarily was to help people live safely in the community. The delivery of care was now being evaluated and improved accordingly to meet more modern standards.

In 1988 we both moved back to the North East and I acquired a post on day duty at St Lukes Hospital in Middlesbrough. We bought a house locally and our travelling days were over as far as moving from one hospital to another went. We had always planned to return home, and the qualifications we had gained gave us the flexibility to do this. At that time there were more vacancies for mental health nurses all over the country, so we were fortunate. I also now had seven years of experience working in different settings, days and nights, on a range of wards from admission to long stay, locked and unlocked. My CV was now looking quite impressive.

We also planned to start a family and one year later our son, Steven, was born. As we say in Yorkshire "I was proud as punch" of becoming a father for the first time. I was working away steadily at the hospital. I was now working on an acute admission ward and was to work in that environment for the next five years.

The 1990's within mental health also heralded more robust Advocacy services for patients to have a stronger voice in the care they received, and also the service delivery overall. This was a ground-breaking move and so far removed from the early eighties approaches. The patients now believed they were being listened to more, and empowerment became a key word. Ex- patients volunteered to support patients receiving treatment. They would attend ward rounds and meetings that could sometimes become formal, quite intimidating forums for the patient.

Who better to provide support than those who had

Sticks and Stones

experience of being in hospital and suffering similar conditions? As nurses we are all advocates for those under our care. The advocacy service provided a more objective support service, for example for those who were being sectioned under the Mental Health Act, as the advocates weren't directly involved in the patient's daily care.

Essentially, going back to the importance of a trusting Nurse/ Patient relationship is the key. If the relationship is strong the nurse may be able to encourage a patient to have treatment, thus avoiding the use of the Mental Health Act to forcibly treat someone lacking insight into their condition. This again has to be put into context. The majority of those I have treated over many years have been treated informally, without the need to use the powers of the Mental Health Act.

The Mental Health Act is used only as a last resort when all other methods have been exhausted. This was to be something I would use later in my awareness-raising in schools and colleges to further shatter the myths of men in white coats using straitjackets to enforce treatment on patients.   It was indeed an exciting time to be in nursing, and changes for the better were coming at a faster pace than ever before.

Sticks and Stones

Chapter 10 – Pastures New

In 1994 my daughter, Laura, was born. As with Steven I was overjoyed. I had always wanted a daughter and my prayers had been answered. I think personally that having children also helps immensely with the empathising process. It touches the heart like nothing else and I cherish both my children. They say you would die for your children and I can understand why. I would for mine. Hopefully that will never be put to the test. As Spike Milligan once said "I'm not afraid of dying, I just don't want to be there when it happens".

Whenever I look at my children I consider the possibility of them ever becoming ill, either mentally or physically, and the care that they would receive. This is the same as with any loved one. We would all like to be treated the same as the next person. This has helped me to stay focused in my work and deliver the highest standard of care to each and every patient. I always think that this person could be my son or my daughter, so how would I expect them to be treated?

Both Teresa and I had contemplated moving over to Ireland to make a fresh start. We would be closer to her family, particularly her mother who was not in good health. I was becoming a bit "burnt out" and needed a fresh challenge. So in

Sticks and Stones

March 1996 we sold our house and moved over to Enniskillen, Co Fermanagh, Teresa's birthplace. We rented a house on a local farm and for a few months enjoyed the break from work and new surroundings. Steven got a place at the local school, Tattygar, which was a small primary school. I got a job working in a local nursing home and Teresa also. Unfortunately the political situation took a turn for the worse with the breakdown of the IRA ceasefire. The Orangemen were also protesting at Drumcree Church which became an international news event for all the wrong reasons. We both began to wonder whether we had made the right decision.

One Saturday night in November I had gone to bed at around midnight and suddenly I heard a bang. It sounded like it was coming from some distance away but was still audible enough. I went outside and all I could hear was a deadly silence for a few minutes, and then the sound of dogs all barking from the surrounding farms. The next day I put the television on and saw the remains of the Killyhevlin hotel near Enniskillen, about 5 miles away, and a reporter explaining how it had been blown up the previous evening by a bomb. The continuity IRA had accepted responsibility. This was too close for comfort. I went outside and noticed one of the side windows had been cracked and decided to drive to the hotel to see for myself the damage. It was extensive and looked like a war zone.

Sticks and Stones

Teresa's aunt and uncle lived on the banks of Loch Erne, and the loch had flooded their garden, such was the impact of the explosion. The hotel had been packed with a wedding reception and one of the staff had noticed a ticking sound coming from a car parked very close to the main door. The fact that the car was parked ridiculously close to the main door had aroused his suspicion, and the ticking confirmed his worse fears. We felt uneasy about staying in Ireland. Our relatives nearby noticed IRA graffiti had been daubed on their shed door, which was 5 miles from the nearest town. This was out in the countryside where very few incidents of this kind ever occurred. It was a very tense and difficult time for everyone in the province and the country was on the brink of civil war. We decided to return to England and start afresh.

Chapter 11 – Returning to England

March 1997 and I was back in England and working for the Trust I had worked for previously in Middlesbrough. I was fortunate to acquire a post on the admission unit as a staff nurse. Two years later I applied for promotion in the form of a Senior Nurse post and I was successful. All my years of training, experience and commitment had paid off and a new challenge was faced. I continued to work within the hospital environment until 2001 when the opportunity arose for me to move into a Community Mental Health Resource Centre. I applied for a post of Senior Nurse in a local centre. I have been there ever since.

In 2002 the Trust started a campaign to positively promote mental health issues locally. It was an anti stigma campaign under the title of the "Passionate People" Campaign. I think this title symbolizes everything. We are a group of people who are passionate about changing society's attitudes towards our services and patients. I liked this concept, and eagerly volunteered to be part of this initiative. The work would involve visiting local schools and colleges to raise awareness and dispel the common myths and misconceptions that surround mental ill health.

I thought that being part of the campaign would provide me with an ideal opportunity to use my many years in nursing, which had at this point

Sticks and Stones

reached twenty-one, to challenge all the myths and stereotypes. I was in a position to put the record straight. I could explain it as it was, from someone who has been in the "business" for long enough to be qualified to do this.

I soon found myself visiting many schools and colleges. I would also visit local libraries, and anywhere else that expressed an interest in understanding more about mental illness. I relished this work. I had a very supportive Manager who allowed me to negotiate the time in which to do this, in addition to my daily duties as a Community Nurse. As a consequence of my own flexibility, and the success of my specific talks, I found myself being asked more and more to go back to certain schools. There became a greater demand to increase my work. I was more than happy to do this, as I also gained a great deal of enjoyment and satisfaction from knowing I was making a difference. I was also meeting many different people from different walks of life than my own. This work became so satisfying.

I felt like I had a new sense of vigour. I was enthused about something as never before. Mental Health promotion in this country has never received the same amount of funding or priority as in other parts of Britain, such as Scotland, where the "See Me" campaign has greatly spread the message and challenged the discrimination. The work I was doing could be replicated in many other areas given the necessary funding to make

Sticks and Stones

a difference in society.

My work was voluntary, and when talking to people from other parts of the country I learnt that our Trusts campaign was way ahead of other organisations in actively addressing stigma. I have been very fortunate indeed to work for an organisation that places emphasis on tackling the inequalities that exist through a specific campaign such as the "Passionate People" campaign.

Our Trusts Public Relations department, which I began to work more closely with, would regularly give me contacts that I could visit. In time I forged useful links and after about a year found myself getting direct phone calls from outside agencies requesting my input. I would always liaise with the Public Relations department to inform them of what I was doing, and they were very supportive of my commitment and enthusiasm to the cause.

On my college visits I would talk to students who were going to chose healthcare as a career. I answered their questions and dispelled some of the commonly held beliefs. I would explain the workings of a community mental health team, how people are referred, and treatment programmes. Self harm by cutting is something that has increased among young people so I would also touch on this, and drug abuse, which has implications on one's mental health, sometimes which can be very long lasting. At a local Library I found myself talking with a colleague to the Library

Sticks and Stones

group, again the theme was mental health promotion and we used the session as an informal question and answer session. Tea and biscuits were on the menu. There were about 12 people in the room of different ages, but mostly elderly.

One lady who would have been in her late sixties or early seventies asked me if people became mentally ill because they were naughty as children. I was temporarily speechless before responding to her question. At that moment I knew that the work myself and many other people do around challenging the myths is so important. I thought that this lady had been carrying that belief inside her mind for many, many, years and it would invariably have influenced her attitude and behaviour towards anyone she deemed to be mentally ill; a sobering thought. Such was the ignorance.

Sticks and Stones

Chapter 12 – A Dark Place

In September 2004 following months of believing I was coping, and deluding myself that stress only affected others less able than myself, reality struck home and I became severely depressed. In hindsight I should have seen it coming, as with the car accident all those years before, but I didn't. I was stressed and depressed, the primary reasons for this being a reaction to a close colleague becoming seriously ill in hospital, and an increased, more demanding workload. All the classic symptoms of depression were there but I couldn't see them. I couldn't see the wood for the trees which happens all to often in depression..

On a personal level I was becoming over-sensitive and self critical. My decision-making became non-existent, and even when I found myself in a position to make a decision I couldn't. Or I would question the decision repeatedly inside my head. Was it the right one? Slowly day by day over a period of months my confidence and ability to function sapped. I have the benefit of hindsight now to realise these concerns, but at the time it was as if I was existing in another world. My reality was so different and alien to everybody else's. Each day became unbearably painful as I persevered and went to work not wanting to let the side down by going off sick. My sense of duty and loyalty went above and beyond anybody else's. It became masochistic.

Sticks and Stones

I didn't spot the warning signs such as panicky feelings in certain situations, and also full blown panic attacks. My concentration was affected and at night I would wake up in the early hours ruminating over things, small things that under normal circumstances should not hamper someone's regular sleep pattern. Insignificant issues took on the proportions of catastrophes. At times I felt as if I was wandering around in another world, separate from reality and closed off from others. With the benefit of hindsight I realise now that this was so wrong, and all I was doing was making life even more difficult for myself, and probably others. In meetings I would feel self-conscious and experience a panic attack. I would feel myself having difficulty breathing and hyperventilating. I would sweat profusely and then as a consequence feel even more self-conscious.

I would go into my small office, close the door, and lock out the world. But this really only brought short term respite. On Friday afternoon when everyone was looking forward to having the weekend off, I still couldn't "switch off", I would wish the weekend away so that I could be back behind my desk on Monday morning. Such was my ridiculous sense of duty and responsibility. Many weekends were lost.

Meetings, where I would ordinarily exude self-confidence, became torturous affairs. At the time in my mind I would wonder if anyone could spot my meltdown, my emotional deterioration. If they

Sticks and Stones

could why were they not saying anything because
it was so out of character for one normally so in
control and confident? I knew the people in the
meetings very well, and would usually feel
comfortable in their presence, but now my
confidence and self esteem was ebbing away,
slowly, like the blood oozing from a dying,
frightened animal. It felt that bad.

The stress had built up over many months, and I
suppressed this by adopting the ridiculous attitude
of 'persevere Lol, and it will all blow over.' Denial
was my mental defence mechanism. It didn't blow
over! In effect it got considerably worse. I was
advised by my Manager at the time to seek
medical help which I did. I then went on sick
leave. I now had time to reflect on my life, and
how I had reached that point.

I was no longer Lol the nurse, but Lol the patient.
The proverbial shoe was now on the other foot.
Interestingly my GP, who was very supportive,
asked me what I would like to be put on the sick
note as the cause of sickness. Would I be happy
with depression? My thoughts about this were,
why not? Surely if I would prefer something else
to be recorded I would be doing the opposite from
what I encouraged others to do, i.e. not feel guilty
or ashamed about having a mental illness. This
would be hypocritical and I certainly didn't want to
play that game.

In hindsight I think everybody else could see that I

Sticks and Stones

was struggling but myself, and this is often the case when we try to mask our true emotions. Hindsight is a great thing of course. I can reflect back now and appreciate that in certain situations I was struggling, but I persevered and tried to look strong to save face. It was akin to being on an emotional roller-coaster ride that I didn't seem to have any control over, a runaway train that was gathering momentum and would crash or derail at some point, with me on board.

I regard this episode as a turning point in my life and an experience that I hope I have learnt much from. I had felt stressed previously as my work is a stressful occupation, but not on this scale, never like this, this was a major wake up call. Here was I, the qualified mental health nurse, who would advise others on a daily basis to talk openly about their problems and not mask their feelings, doing the exact opposite. I was a hypocrite. In many ways I was not unlike many others in my profession who do not believe they will ever encounter stress. Or feel that this is somehow beneath them.

Some in my own profession talk about their own stress and mental health in hushed tones, as if these are words they do not feel comfortable using. It has been like this in all the years I have nursed but I do sense a sea change coming, and hopefully this will bring more acceptance and understanding. Many think they are untouchable, but they are not. I can vouch for that. Many

Sticks and Stones

believe they are too strong and insightful because they have to be always seen as the carers, the professionals who must be in control at all times. Again the stigma aspect rears its ugly head. It's the "them and us" scenario again. I should have known better. No excuses.

Following a three month break I returned to work energised and feeling much better for the rest. I was looking forward to returning and getting back into the work routine again. I enjoy my work and had missed my colleagues and patients and the routine of going to work. I now had to be more aware of my own stress vulnerability level, and not allow myself to ride on the runaway train again. I had to be more insightful as to what keeps me well and what doesn't. It was important for me to understand my limitations. The lesson was learnt and it had been a hard one to learn.

I was touched by all the cards I received from well wishers, staff and patients, on my return to work. I had been prescribed Fluoxetine, better known as Prozac by my GP, and my mood started to lift. I continued to do all the other things so important when fighting depression such as talking to close friends and having a balanced routine that included activity. In my case this was squash and the gym which are both therapeutic for my mental health. I would also continue to spend time with my family and do enjoyable simple things that I would have struggled to do previously.

Sticks and Stones

Not long after returning to work I became involved in an initiative by the Department of Health. This was a project that aimed to define what a positive emotional experience is like for patients, and how their experiences of using services can be enhanced. Historically much of the emphasis within the healthcare system has focused on the practical issues, such as ward layout and the environment, and physical interventions. This project was to focus on the more personal emotional aspects of care. I volunteered to be part of the National Practitioners Forum to help to define what is a positive experience and help to create a more patient led NHS. The other group members, with the exception of myself and another man, were mostly from the Primary Care setting and I viewed this as a way of representing the Secondary Mental Health setting. After all it is just as important to have the needs of those with mental illness addressed in hospital or the community, as it is the patients using general health care facilities. My remit therefore was to look at ways I could enhance this approach within my own workplace.

Ideas were discussed around areas such as in-patient admission wards and having a dedicated nurse to welcome patients and carers to generally ease any worries they have of going into hospital. It is one thing to fill in a form or questionnaire to measure how you feel you are being treated but equally important to have the 'human touch' of being offered a cup of tea, and greeted by

Sticks and Stones

someone with a smile on their face. These are
small often ignored issues, but do impact on
someone's confidence, sense of feeling
appreciated, and ease when going into an
environment they are not familiar with. If I was to
visit a friend or relative on the ward I would like to
be treated with courtesy and respect and be
reassured. We all should expect that at the very
least. The aims of the group were to look at what
often small steps can be taken to facilitate this
process and make any experience of using NHS
services better. In a nutshell it involved going
back to basics in our approaches to patients and
their families.

Over the course of a year I attended two meetings
at the Department of Health in London. At the
meetings we all shared ideas around how we
could improve the patient and relative
experiences within our different work areas. There
were about twenty of us in the focus group. I felt
proud and privileged to represent mental health
services in this forum, more so because only two
of us represented the mental health services
nationally in this specific group. The final
document outlining what areas have been
improved was titled "Now I Feel Tall" and was
released in December 2005. For my part, along
with a few colleagues, I arranged a training day for
all the administration staff within the locality to
share ideas and look at ways of improving our
services.

Chapter 13 – A New Campaign

The media play an important role in ensuring that fair, balanced coverage of issues relating to mental illness is carried out. Unfortunately this isn't always the case. Sensationalism by the media has been very damaging towards those who are mentally ill through the use of derogatory language and exaggerated viewpoints. These usually portray people with mental illness as being dangerous, unpredictable, and usually needing to be locked away, "out of harm's way". This sensationalism and distortion of the truth seems to sell newspapers, and the more exaggerated the facts and lies, the more the papers will sell.

The SHIFT Government campaign to tackle stigma and discrimination surrounding mental illness started in 2004 under the heading "From here to Equality". Shift is part of the Governments Care Services Improvement Partnership (CSIP). It is a five year campaign aimed at tackling stigma that surrounds mental illness in all areas of society. Part of the campaign was the setting up of the "Speakers Bureau" which specifically focuses on addressing negative media coverage of mental illness.

The Bureau is made up entirely of people who have personal experiences of mental illness. They are willing to share their experiences with the media as part of the awareness raising process.

Sticks and Stones

Who better to inform the media than those who have had personal experiences of mental ill-health? I was very interested upon hearing about this initiative so I offered to help by sharing my own experiences with the aim of helping others to understand more. I also thought that my own experiences would have the added bonus of speaking as both a qualified mental health nurse, and a sufferer of depression. I could relate to my own personal experiences, whilst at the same time dispel some of the myths about treatment, hospitals, conditions, and so forth. My openness and honesty may help others within my own profession to do like-wise. My own episode left me feeling more insightful and certainly more empathic. In December 2005 I headed to Manchester to be trained to deal with the media in our bureau work.

I shared a room with like-minded individuals, all with a yearning to redress the imbalance of criminalisation and discrimination by the media. We were all trained on the day by John Morrell, a very distinguished ex-journalist with a very impressive CV. John was what I would describe as a consummate professional.   He had his own Public Relations consultancy and was a passionate supporter of charitable causes. Sadly John has now passed away, but having only known him for a short while I will remember him as a very caring and humble man. He was so polished in his approach, and his years of journalistic experience came through. John will be

Sticks and Stones

sadly missed. At the end of a very exhausting day we all felt more knowledgeable and confident about any future dealings with the press.

I was excited about having a unique opportunity to deliver, through the media, my strong convictions around challenging stigma. I believed also that as a so-called "professional" I had a duty to do this as part of the overall mental health promotion strategy. One of my first assignments was to take part in a radio interview with Matthew Davies, a well-known local DJ on BBC Radio Cleveland. The aim was to look at depression, its signs and symptoms, and explain about my own particular experience. When asked to do this I was more than happy to oblige. I was made to feel welcome in the studio, and the interview took place on the early morning show at around 8 am. The questions I was asked focused on depression and medication and the efficacy of this. It had followed recent research indicating a rise in stress related illnesses.

Stress had overtaken back problems as the most commonly diagnosed reason for sickness on prescriptions, so my views were sought on the possible reasons for this. Matthew has my utmost respect because he had done his homework and was very knowledgeable about the subject. He told me about serotonin and dopamine chemicals being depleted causing depression, and recent research at that time encouraging more people to eat bananas. As a result of the interview a

Sticks and Stones

number of people approached me saying they had listened to the interview and felt it was brave of me to share my own personal experiences, particularly because I was a mental health nurse.

For my part I believe that regardless of who I am, and what I do, the opportunity arose to spread the word and I was flattered to have been asked to do this. How could I possibly refuse? Only by more people speaking out, particularly within my own profession, will the stigma be addressed.

I found myself receiving more requests to visit schools and colleges locally. Each time the phone rang with a request I did my utmost to oblige. I was enjoying my new-found anti stigma role immensely and accepted every challenge with gusto. It was interesting to meet new people, and visit places that I wouldn't have ordinarily have had the opportunity to visit. All of this was in addition to my full time role as a Senior Nurse and all the responsibilities this entailed.

At times it was difficult to oblige every request, but I tried my utmost to help out as I didn't want to let anyone down. Sometimes this meant working in my own time, but this was a choice I made. I wasn't being forced to do it, I enjoyed the work so much I wanted to do it. The local newspaper, The Evening Gazette, based in Middlesbrough, soon became aware of my passion to positively promote all issues relating to mental health. In the summer of 2005 I started to engage more with the Gazette,

Sticks and Stones

with the view to building up positive links with the journalists and forging a closer working relationship.

I was still liaising closely with our Public Relations department, but to some degree I was now given more autonomy. It is common knowledge that so much criminalisation and sensationalism is perpetuated by the press in relation to mental illness. We are all too familiar with phrases such as "looney" and "nutter" being casually used by some of the national newspapers. My aim was simple. If I could de-stigmatize mental illness through the local press, peoples' perceptions would be challenged and maybe even changed. I could tell it as it is, put the record straight as someone with many years of experience as a qualified mental health clinician. I would certainly give it my best shot.

I began by answering questions around maintaining mental health for the occasional Gazette article. Before long I became a recognisable contact for journalists wanting some more specific information, such as signs and symptoms of certain conditions, and treatment programmes. For the Gazette there was the specialist factor of being a qualified mental health nurse of many years experience opening the doors to a local "asylum". I started submitting my personal views through a section called "I Can Do That" which highlighted health issues in general, and the different conditions both physical and

Sticks and Stones

mental that affect us all. All my personal views and ideas were vetted by our Public Relations Department who were very pleased that I was offering to positively promote our services. We shared the same vision of course.

By having my articles printed as part of a collective piece that looks at health in general the demystifying process began. I would stress the important correlation between physical and mental health, and how they cannot be separated, one will affect the other. Therefore in order to maintain both to the best of our abilities we must look after them both equally and view them as two sides of the same coin and very much interlinked.

I hold strong views around what is right and wrong and in particular the stigmatization of our service users and services. At the moment I am concerned about the rise of so called "reality TV" programmes and their depiction of the mentally ill. At times I have watched programmes that allow people to open themselves up to ridicule by the panel of judges and the audience. This doesn't sit comfortably with me and I wonder how many of these people are in fact mentally ill and unaware of the situation they have found themselves in. I accept that sometimes people will crave the limelight and the attention that these kind of programmes provide. However, when observing some people I believe, as someone with many years of experience and knowledge, that they are being exploited for the entertainment of the mass

Sticks and Stones

population and that worries me greatly. Are we becoming a society where it is acceptable to ridicule for the sake of amusement?

There is a lack of respect and tolerance in many sections of society, and we are faced daily with news stories of "happy slapping" incidents and unprovoked assaults, often leading to death. Knife crime is on the increase and we seem to have lost many of our youth population to anti-social behaviour and criminality. I feel that TV programmes have a responsibility to promote respect and consideration of all people and not target a section of society such as the mentally ill and make them scapegoats.

In time my links with the Gazette increased, and I negotiated with my contacts the submission of more regular articles to spread the message. I intended to make the articles more thought-provoking for people to question their own prejudices, attitudes, and behaviours. I am indebted to the Gazette, particularly journalists Marie Turbill and Marie Levy, for affording me this opportunity to positively promote mental health issues. I have submitted the articles regularly, and have appeared in the health supplement. I am grateful to the Gazette for giving me permission to reproduce them in this book, all the articles are appended at the back.

Every year the Trust that I work for holds an annual awards event. This is to recognise good

Sticks and Stones

practices and give credit to those who have "gone the extra mile" and positively promoted the organisation through their endeavours. I was extremely flattered to have been nominated by a colleague for my anti stigma work which won the first prize in the 2006 "Tackling Inequalities" section. This was recognition for all the hard work I had carried out and a great motivating factor for me.

Through my work I strongly believe I am reaching people by encouraging reflection and debate around certain attitudes and behaviours. The awards ceremony took place in a local hotel, Gisborough Hall, and it was also inspiring to meet colleagues and service users who share the same dedication and passion for their different projects. A fabulous night was had by all.

I continued to work within my clinical role, and tried wherever possible to assist with any requests from the Speakers Bureau, even if this meant, which was often the case, working within my own time outside of work. As with the school project, I was able to meet many people who inspired me with their enthusiasm and dedication. I continued to take on each and every request with relish.

I arrived at work one morning in mid November 2006 and opened my emails and letters. To my surprise, and absolute delight, I had been nominated by a colleague, Simon, from the Public Relations Department, for the CSIP Positive

Sticks and Stones

Practice Awards 2006. I had been highly commended for the "Leadership in Promoting Anti Stigma and Discrimination" award.

The ceremony would take place at Chelsea Football club, and myself and a guest would be invited to attend the ceremony, which included dinner, travel expenses, and accommodation. To say I was surprised would have been an understatement. I felt deeply moved and humbled. I was appreciative to Simon for his nomination and also for the recognition CSIP had afforded me.

The ceremony took place on 23rd November 2006 and I headed down to London with Teresa, my wife, as my guest. The night was to be one of the nicest evenings I have ever spent and I felt privileged to meet so many ordinary people like myself, who all share the same passion for positively promoting mental health issues, and challenging inequality. Here I felt comfortable among people I respected for their honesty, integrity and strength. Many have overcome adversity from one source or another and by doing this have given hope to many others who find themselves without a voice and disenfranchised.

At the start of the evening, which was attended by around a hundred people, I was asked to stand and receive an ovation from all the invited guests and nominees. At this point I concentrated my mind on what I had achieved, and where I had

Sticks and Stones

come from. The journey had been long but well worth it.

From such humble beginnings here was I, a working class Northern lad, who had defied all the odds. Through sheer endeavour, determination and resilience I had made a real impact in my native North East which was now being recognised and rewarded Nationally. I believed I was putting the North East on the map for all the right reasons. This part of the North East is all too often given a negative press through the media, one that it certainly doesn't merit. This isn't helped by the child abuse inquiry of the late 1980's which made national headlines and polarised this part of the country for all the wrong reasons. Mud sticks unfortunately. There are many decent, hard-working and caring people in this region, down to earth people who would always help in time of need, and would give you their last penny if necessary. Also people like myself who are committed to tackling the inequalities that exist within this region. The framed certificate now sits proudly in my office, a daily reminder of the evening, and the ongoing campaign I strive to promote. It is a great motivator for me and something I am very proud of.

Sticks and Stones

Chapter 14 – The Huge Bag of Worries

In June 2006 I was approached by a lady who also works within the Trust and who, like myself, had a passion for mental health promotion. Her name is Marjorie, and she wanted to discuss a creative idea she had around positively promoting mental health in primary schools. This was through the use of a 'Story Sacks' approach. We arranged to meet to discuss her idea to explore whether I could be of help in developing this within local primary schools.

A story sack is a large cloth bag containing a good quality storybook with supporting materials, such as puppets, soft toys and a game to stimulate reading, language and numeric activities. There is usually a cassette tape with the story recorded onto it so the children can follow along and act out. Story Sacks were developed by Neil Griffiths, formally a head teacher in Swindon who went onto direct the National Support Project for Story Sacks on behalf of the Basic Skills Agency. The initiative spread to schools, pre-schools and libraries throughout the country. They are designed to help adults share books with children in a way that is positive, theatrical, special, interactive and fun. Marjorie's idea was that this could be extended to the subject of mental health which is not on the national curriculum.

Our meeting was very fruitful. Between us we

Sticks and Stones

explored the idea of using an interactive story sack approach within local primary schools to raise awareness of the detrimental impact bullying has on a child's emotional health and well-being. By doing this we could also de-stigmatize mental health services and service users. It was a two pronged approach.

There are a number of books written for children around bullying, and encouraging specific techniques to address this. Marjorie and I both sat and read a number of these to give us some ideas.

The one book that immediately captured our imagination for its beautiful graphics and narrative was "The Huge Bag of Worries" written by Virginia Ironside and illustrated by Frank Rodgers. It told the story of a young girl who was very upset because she was carrying all her worries around in a large sack that was wearing her down both physically and emotionally. We contacted the publishers to confirm it would be acceptable to use the book for our work. They held the copyright and told us they were more than happy to support this. Many schools already use the book as a reading aid, but our approach specifically relating the book to bullying and mental health is unique.

Our plan was to both deliver this on a Power Point whiteboard display whilst Marjorie read the story. In order to capture the children's imagination and help them understand how worries can be a

Sticks and Stones

burden, the programme uses worries that are physical in appearance; some are soft and furry and easy to resolve, whilst others are heavy and rough and can take longer to deal with. The huge bag of worries made by Marjorie is a very colourful sack which steadily gets bigger and bigger when the worries are added to the bag. In order for the children to understand how mental health and physical health work together the children have the opportunity to carry the bag around and see for themselves how it slows them down and gets in the way. The main focus was around bullying, and encouraging the children to accept that it is normal to have worries and important to share them, particularly heavy worries, such as bullying.

It is also a fact of life that many of these young children will have family members who will suffer from mental illness, and we hope that this simple approach explains that everyone has mental health and that they learn to treat those people they recognise as having mental ill-health with respect and understanding; often these children are already young carers.

At the end of the day we would all congregate in the playground where the children release the helium balloons which represent Jenny's worries, the children count down from ten to zero and then they are released one by one which is how we deal with our worries. We hope this gives a powerful symbolic message to the children which leaves them uplifted.

Sticks and Stones

Initially we approached Ravensworth Junior School in Normanby to see if they would be open to us trialling it there. This is Marjorie's son's school. Kevin Skelton, the Head Teacher, was open to us trialling it there, he explained that his own mother had worked as an Occupational Therapist at St Lukes which is the local Mental Health Hospital within our Trust, so he was empathetic to our aims. The school understood we did not normally work with children and met with us prior to talk about the approach and practical considerations and how the session would run. The day at Ravensworth on 5th June 2006 seemed to go well, and we were pleased when Kevin Skelton invited us to present our idea at the local SEAL (Social and Emotional Aspects of Learning) conference later in the month. SEAL is a resource that has been launched throughout primary schools throughout the Country, and all the primary schools within Redcar and Cleveland were meeting to provide feedback on the different ways they had implemented its use. Our target audience could not have been better.

Again, I viewed this as a way of positively promoting mental health services and raising my own profile locally within schools. I was building on the already very useful links I had forged with local schools. As a consequence of the positive feedback from the conference, we soon found ourselves arranging input into a number of local primary schools, initially piloting the programme in 10 schools, then evaluating the feedback from

Sticks and Stones

teachers and pupils. I have to say that the programme in its essence is the same as it was in the beginning, but the honest feedback from teachers was invaluable and helped us improve our delivery and style, which helps other schools to benefit at a later stage, so our thanks to all those schools who participated.

To date we have visited over 20 schools in many diverse areas of the region. This work is ongoing and our aim is to eventually deliver this in other areas building on the success of the programme locally. We have been enthused by the response to our programme and from the feedback we have received. It is clear to me that there is a need to significantly increase mental health awareness in schools. There remain concerning issues, bullying being just one such issue, that need to be robustly addressed. Our programme is a simple, but equally highly effective way of approaching the subject of mental health.

Many people who access mental health services do so because they have a diagnosis of depression. In quite a number of cases this can be attributed to unresolved issues in childhood that have seriously impacted on self esteem and worth. Often these issues can be attributed to bullying at school which wasn't addressed at the time. Our programme reinforces the message of sharing worries. The outcome of not dealing with worries can cause problems in later life once the child has reached adulthood. We also reach the

Sticks and Stones

teaching staff and the parents through the programme, thereby positively promoting mental health and well-being. The balloon release at the end always prompts questions by the parents collecting their children to find out what the children have been doing. We always send home a letter to the parents explaining what their child has learnt and what steps everyone can take to maintain their own mental health; another audience we may not have targeted but through the school's willingness to let us go in we have reached.

Our school work was gaining momentum and we were now becoming easily recognised locally as the couple who were more than willing to visit any school to spread our campaign message. Our huge bag of worries was being dragged from school to school. At each school we met many excited children, all eager to see what was inside this colourful sack. We derived as much pleasure as the children in delivering our story. The teachers also appreciated our input, and we feel learnt much about their own mental health, and ways in which this can be maintained.

NIMHE (National Institute for Mental Health in England) publicised our creative project as a positive practise initiative in their Mental Health Promotion newsletter. This helped us to increase awareness of our innovative approach nationally.

The momentum of the project had been greatly

Sticks and Stones

boosted when we were short-listed to attend the Tees, Esk & Wear Valleys NHS Trust "Making a Difference 2007" awards ceremony for the "Tackling Stigma and Promoting Social Inclusion" category. Both Marjorie and myself work for the Trust and we knew there was a lot of competition as the Trust had recently merged and is the second largest mental health and learning disability Trust in England. We could not have been more pleased when we won the category for our "Story Sack" approach, indeed we had caught the eye of our Trust Board and key people who are now supporting us is progressing this approach into other areas, including Teesside University.

I have to admit receiving these awards has been flattering and very complimentary, but the truth is that I am hoping that these can be used as leverage to open doors into other areas to tackle the stigma that still exists, as this is my real passion and what drives me forward.

Sticks and Stones

Chapter 15 – The Wider Community

In January 2007 I was asked if I would do a presentation around how the stigmatizing of mental health impacts on those who have mental illness in employment, at the CSIP "Action on Stigma" conference to be held in York. The target audience were around 200 employers. I was asked to give three anonymous examples of people who I have known within mental health services who have either been discriminated against, or are reluctant to apply for jobs because they feel stigmatised.

Sadly it is a well known fact that many people do not even apply for jobs fearing that as soon as mental illness is mentioned their chances of getting the job will be reduced. This then becomes a self fulfilling prophecy. The aim of the conference was to encourage more understanding and acceptance within employment.

This was to be the first time I had ever presented to such a large audience, and to some degree I didn't prepare myself as well as I could have. I was very nervous as I walked up to the podium, though afterwards it was fed back to me that I didn't look nervous at all. I was told I appeared very composed. We all know looks can be deceptive. Maybe I should have chosen acting as a career? As the old saying goes "fail to prepare, prepare to fail"

Sticks and Stones

I decided to speak from the heart, with the hope of getting the message across. It worked. The audience liked what I had said and it touched their hearts too. Nothing will drive the message home more effectively I believe than real life experiences. I was speaking from the heart, recounting real life anonymous experiences, rather than reading from a textbook, and they seemed to empathise and identify with this very well.

The feedback was very positive and my self esteem and confidence was further boosted. More importantly the message was delivered to a large audience of employers, who hopefully will recall my words whenever they are in the position of interviewing someone with a mental illness. They will look beyond the label and see the person rather than the illness. This was to be the main thrust of the message. Most people who have a diagnosed mental health condition want to work and yet the majority are not in work. This doesn't add up of course. The reasons for this can be related to the stigma they experience or the perceived stigma they will experience, as well as their own personal condition preventing them from working.

Not long after this I was asked, again through the Speakers Bureau, if I would share my own experience of depression with Jim Pollard, who is the editor for the Male Health website. They were doing a feature on depression aimed at education around the common symptoms, and also touching on medication, its efficacy and side effects. I was more than happy to oblige.

I continued to submit articles for the local newspaper, The Evening Gazette, each time trying to look at different areas of healthcare to address, but underpinning all these was the stigma message. This was the main message I wanted to deliver. It was becoming my own mantra. In June 2007 I was asked to take part in another Radio Cleveland interview with Matthew Davies, the subject was depression again. Once again I was impressed with the research Matthew had done into the topic. Through sheer determination and drive I was now working almost full time in my anti stigma role. My name was now becoming synonymous locally with the anti stigma campaign. I cannot remember when I ever felt as passionate about a subject.

In September 2007 further recognition for my anti-stigma work came when I was asked if I would like to work on a part time basis to develop an anti stigma approach in local employment, and also build on the school story sacks project. I jumped at the chance. It meant I could dedicate more time to something I enjoy immensely, and also gave me the opportunity to work with Marjorie in a more structured and timely way. This was to be funded through the Healthy Communities Programme looking at emotional health and well-being awareness. It is a one year project.

Sticks and Stones

To coincide with World mental health week, which takes place every October, I had prepared myself for getting involved in some promotion work. This tends to be the busiest week of the year as far as the mental health awareness and promotion calendar go. I had pieced together a small stigma stand to exhibit at a local library in Grangetown in Middlesbrough with the intention of highlighting the different ways of addressing stigma in society. I would highlight the different ways I had spread the message locally. The library had numerous other activities and displays all spreading the same message of promoting tolerance, respect and understanding. Holding the exhibition in a local well attended library ensured quite a few people would come in and look at the different stands and take part in other activities that had also been arranged.

I had also been asked by CSIP if I would take part in a conference at Hardwick Hall in Sedgefield, County Durham, to look at stigma within employment, and share my own personal experiences as a mental health nurse, and also as someone who has experienced depression. The conference would also focus on what can be done to support people with mental health problems in the workplace. Both events were to take place on the same day. I couldn't let this opportunity slip away. I decided I would attend the conference, which went on until about 2.30pm and then go to Middlesbrough and man my little stand in the library. Problem solved!

Sticks and Stones

The conference was an opportunity for me to talk to the employers present about my own depressive episode, and how I managed it. I was nervous, as always on these occasions. I would explain my own experience and the support I received to encourage others to look at what systems can be put in place to help others. I was even more nervous on this occasion because I was going to be explicit and open about my own personal experience to members of my own Trust, as well as to the employers who had been invited. Some of the people in the audience I knew and were probably not aware of my depression four years previously. It is a very large organisation and I have worked with many people over many years.

As I started to speak I glanced at everyone wondering what they were thinking, particularly those who were not aware of my illness and may have perceived me to be an easy going sort of guy who never appeared to be particularly stressed. I had masked it well. My slot was to be twenty minutes with questions afterwards about how we maintain our mental health, and specifically how I have been since my episode. As always on these occasions the twenty minutes flew by.

As I was speaking and looking at each person I was getting the odd nod or smile of support which is always helpful when delivering a speech, especially one I feel is so personal. It wasn't quite like reliving my depressive episode but it did

Sticks and Stones

open up some small wounds. This was such a public arena in which to do so. Here was I almost opening up my soul and disclosing information that was so personal and intimate; information that would usually only be disclosed during therapy. I did hold back somewhat but still endeavoured to get the most salient points across without making it some kind of psychotherapeutic counselling session. I spoke about the support I had received which is so important, and I also wanted to make it a positive speech to highlight that there is life after illness. For any of those who have suffered mental illness including depression, we must all have aspirations and hope in order to move forward. This was something that I also had to stress. Yes, I had suffered, but I has also recovered, and there is every reason to believe that if I look after myself well from now on I will never relapse again. Time will tell.

When we become nervous we often experience pressure of speech. I could talk for Great Britain in the Olympics if I had to, if it became an event. I was conscious of getting the points across without rambling on and becoming incoherent. I took deep breaths and pauses and became very focused on my breathing and voice tone. When we are nervous our voice tone becomes higher pitched and I was conscious of this not becoming the case.

I survived. More people within the organisation now became aware of my own personal

Sticks and Stones

experiences. Previously many would have thought that my work promoting mental health wasn't such a personal effort, but more a job that I was being paid to do. They could now see that it was much more than that. It had become almost my 'raison d'etre'. Afterwards a couple of people came up to me and congratulated me and thanked me for my honesty. I appreciated that.

Both Marjorie and I continued our school project and were enthused each time by the positive reactions of the teachers and pupils. I never cease to be amazed by the reactions of the children. At each school we were also building good bonds with the staff, and it gave us an insight into the stresses and pressures the teachers face daily.

I continued to work between my clinical role and mental health promotion. My son Steven had also been successful in acquiring a place at Teesside University to start his mental health Diploma training. He was eighteen. We now had three nurses in the family! In March a request came through from Ben Furner at the SHIFT Speakers Bureau, to ask if I would be happy to take part in the BBC Headroom campaign. This was all part of a new BBC campaign to positively promote Mental Health and Well-being through the media. Headroom is an ambitious 2 year campaign to encourage people to look after both their emotional and physical health. As usual I was more than happy to take part. This would involve

Sticks and Stones

a 2 minute video blog looking at my own episode of depression, and what I do now to stay well. Frightening stuff in some ways, as once more I would be disclosing personal information about myself. The video would then be seen at exhibitions, BBC 3, the internet and in libraries across the country to raise awareness. Ameneh Enayat, a freelance journalist, came all the way up from London and we filmed one sunny afternoon in March 2008 here in Guisborough, North Yorkshire, my home town. I am pleased with the result. I look forward to seeing what impact it has within the wider community and nationally.

Sticks and Stones

Chapter 16- The Future

In September of this year I will be 48, which means in 7 years time I will be eligible to retire from the health service on a full pension. My mother used to say we shouldn't wish away our lives but it is something I am looking forward to greatly. By then I will have been working in the Health Service for 37 years. I rest my case. Throughout this period I have seen many changes, mostly positive I am pleased to say. I have seen the demise of the padded cell, not before time, and the greater promotion of advocacy, empowerment and patients rights. I have also seen the discontinuation of medications that caused more problems due to their side effect profile, and the introduction of more therapeutic medications with fewer side effects and better efficacy. Home treatment interventions are now available in addition to the traditional inpatient admission as the only option available for treatment. This ensures that more people are treated within their home environment, near to their relatives and loved ones which has proven to be more beneficial in the long term. I also believe we are more client centred in our approach to care than ever before, and we are more accountable for our practises also.

The emphasis now is more on promotion of well-being and wellness as opposed to treatment, prevention rather than cure. In the early days of

Sticks and Stones

the seventies the emphasis was more on medication and treatment within the hospital confines. Much has changed. The holistic approaches of today concentrate on the physical, psychological, social and spiritual aspects of care, recognising that the person's needs can be more fully addressed looking at all these areas. It isn't only about giving someone a tablet to make them feel better, it is more proactive and educational, teaching people how to lead a healthy lifestyle both physically and mentally; empowerment and choice, negotiation and collaboration of care required, rather than the old days of custodial and wholly prescriptive care.

Secondary care services, such as mental health teams, now work more closely with the Primary Care Services, and this is also beneficial in helping to remove the stigma. Patients are now termed Service Users. Healthcare is addressed with both physical and psychological needs being acknowledged as working in correlation rather than separately.

In all honesty sometimes I feel like a Nursing dinosaur, especially when I meet students and qualified staff who weren't even born when I started out. My memory isn't as sharp as it used to be which is either a sign of ageing or taking too much on. Or both. I have had to become computer efficient over recent years as the changes have meant much more computer technology with electronic records replacing the

Sticks and Stones

old paper case-notes. This didn't come easy, as I was more familiar with writing everything down in old 'Kardex' systems, but I became adept eventually. I don't think I could function without my emails now. I still have many years of experience behind me, and thankfully most students and junior staff treat me with respect and acknowledge this. I hope that I inspire them with my attitude and approach towards tackling stigma and promoting the rights of service users. I would like to see more young people becoming involved in challenging inequalities so that when I do hang up my boots (or white coat as some would lead us to believe) others will take my place and continue the fight.

My loyalty, commitment, and most importantly client centred approach remains after all this time. I will always support the underdog because I have been there myself. I have personally experienced stigma through my father's illness, so understand how this touches one's inner emotions. Empathy comes easier when you have personally suffered from mental illness and you believe you can truly put yourself in someone else's shoes. Once the client centred focus has gone it is time for me to follow as this is at the core of being a good nurse. Our plans are to hopefully retire to our second home, a small bungalow in beautiful County Fermanagh and only a stones throw from Loch Erne. In the meantime who knows what fate has in store. I will continue to develop the Huge Bag of Worries in local primary schools and hopefully

Sticks and Stones

further afield. We want to spread the good work. Other schools in Middlesbrough have expressed an interest, and we are looking to trialling this in a school that has a population from a different cultural background where mental health is even more taboo. Mental health is not recognised within some minority communities and as such the stigma, ignorance, and social exclusion, is even more apparent than in mainstream communities.

I am grateful to my colleague Marjorie for supporting me when we deliver the programme. It can be physically and emotionally draining but extremely rewarding to see the faces of the young children, and hear their hopes, dreams and aspirations. Today's children are tomorrow's adults who will influence societies attitudes and opinions. Marjorie's passion and work ethic keeps me inspired and motivated. This is why I enjoy our working relationship and the chemistry between us so much. Sometimes my moods fluctuate and I wonder if I am relapsing again, I still have a tendency not to say "no" as much as I should, and consequently my lack of assertiveness results in my taking on more than I can cope with sometimes. I think I am probably being over sensitive to my mental health on occasions, but I have visited that dark place before and wouldn't like to make a return journey, if that can be avoided. I can identify the trigger signs much sooner now, so feel better prepared. It has to be said that doing too little can be just as harmful to our mental health as we all need a bit of stress to

Sticks and Stones

release adrenalin which gives us a 'feel good factor'. Everyone is different, we all have a different 'stress vulnerability level', it's a case of each individual understanding what their own stress level is. It's all a very fine balancing act and I have learnt to balance well.

I will continue my SHIFT Speakers Bureau work as this gives me so much satisfaction in its diversity. Sometimes I feel restricted, working within a small rural area, and the bureau work allows me to visit other places, meet other people and spread the word further afield. Opening my inner soul for all the world to see must seem masochistic to some, and difficult to comprehend, but hey it beats working in a scampi factory! And I can still feel my fingers! Employment locally is an area that Marjorie and I will keep addressing to raise awareness and tackle stigma. Here in the North East we have a large heavy industry presence where a macho culture exists. These are particular areas where we want to spread the word. I will continue my bi-monthly newspaper articles with the Evening Gazette for as long as they are happy for me to do so. It encourages me when people comment about what they have read. I will wait to see what the reaction is from the Video Nation blog. I am expecting those who are not familiar with my depressive episode 4 years ago to approach me and make some comment, especially in my own profession where much stigma work still needs to be done. I cannot at this moment in time see myself retiring completely

Sticks and Stones

when I reach 55. I would like to do some voluntary work, this would have to be around mental health promotion as I feel as passionate about this now as ever before. I suppose after all this time it must run through my veins.

If my father saw me now I would like to think he would be proud of me and what I have achieved. It has been a long and hard struggle and I have had to overcome many barriers along the way, both personally and professionally. His lasting memory may be of a young boy with tears in his eyes and a look of confusion and bewilderment. So much water has now gone under the bridge and that was such a long time ago. My sincere wish is that when my children become adults they will live in a society that shows more tolerance and respect towards everyone, and in particular the mentally-ill.

Sticks and Stones

ARTICLES PUBLISHED BY THE PRESS

(22/8/05 – Evening Gazette)

"HE must have been insane!" and "Nobody in their right minds could have done that!" How many times have we heard these sentences, usually in response to having read an eye catching headline relating to a particularly vicious crime.

Why is it that we automatically assume the perpetrator must be suffering from a mental illness? The statistics tell a different story.

Less than 5% of people who kill have a diagnosis of mental illness, 95% of serious crime is carried out by people who are not mentally ill.

We stigmatise and socially exclude those within society who experience mental health problems. These people are also more likely to experience discrimination in the areas of physical health care, employment, housing and the criminal justice system.

Negative media coverage and stigmatising only serves to compound the situation and it can be a vicious circle of exclusion.

Sticks and Stones

One in four of the population experience mental health problems, it does not discriminate; it could affect anyone at any time.

Mental illness is stigmatised in all cultures, this is more so in the developed countries.

I work as a senior nurse within mental health and I dedicate as much time as I can towards the positive promotion of mental health.

I dispel the myths and challenge the stigma. I visit schools and colleges to present the facts, not the fiction.

Contrary to negative stereotyping I do not wear a long white coat and neither do my colleagues.

It has been extremely useful when talking to the pupils to receive feedback from them about their own perceptions of mental illness and how this relates to reality.

Talking to children about my own experiences and shattering preconceived ideas doesn't always improve my popularity; younger children, once they realise that stories from within the walls of "the asylum" do not resemble the exaggerated sensationalised TV depiction, can soon become disillusioned.

Building a rapport with children creates trust and encourages open discussions.

Sticks and Stones

Teenagers identify with pressure and stress, this can be experienced as a result of taking exams and peer pressure.

Once a rapport has developed barriers come down and personal issues are raised. "A person I know cuts himself and he seems to be depressed," confided one pupil who was obviously concerned. My immediate thought was, is this student speaking about himself and feeling stigmatised by disclosing such sensitive information? He asked me for advice on how to deal with this kind of behaviour, and who would be the most suitable person for his friend (or himself) to approach. His disclosure opened up a debate around the subject of self harm. Other pupils also related stories about 'friends' who have experienced emotional distress and anguish.

Fortunately more information is now available for all age groups to inform and raise awareness of mental illness.
My school visits play a minor role in the national campaigns to de-stigmatise mental illness.
Better understanding and more tolerance of people who experience mental health problems should be an objective for everyone.

Sticks and Stones

(21/11/05 – Evening Gazette)

In the last edition of I Can Do That I explained the work I do in schools and colleges to dispel the myths that surround mental illness.

Thus far all the feedback I have received has been very encouraging. By recounting my own personal experiences, covering many years as a psychiatric nurse, the proverbial cloak of mystery that shrouds mental illness has been lifted.

By promoting mental illness in a positive light, my aim is to challenge existing negative stereotypes.

Barriers still need to be removed, and more social acceptance and inclusion of those who experience mental health problems is required within society.

When using our services, the importance of improving a patient's overall emotional experience cannot be underestimated. Patients ought to feel that their emotional needs are being addressed; these are wide ranging, from feeling safe and reassured to being listened to and valued.

In times of crisis, and when under stress, we would all wish to be treated with respect and understanding. As a member of staff my own emotional needs will not differ from those of the patients in my care. Therefore being aware of my own emotional needs is important when addressing the emotional needs of my patients. If

Sticks and Stones

a patient's care is of a high quality, and they feel that their emotional needs are being acknowledged and positively addressed, trust in using our services is further enhanced.

I feel this will also continue to challenge negative misconceptions already associated with mental illness. Patients who use mental health services will be at their most vulnerable and because of this their emotions will be heightened. It therefore remains imperative that emotional experiences at this time are positive experiences.

My nursing career covers 25 years. Over this period of time I have been reassured by the many positive changes that have been made within psychiatric nursing. Major improvements have been carried out in relation to the environment within hospitals and community mental health centres. Gone are the endless polished corridors, usually associated with clichéd films depicting "asylums" and custodial care.

More emphasis is now placed on creating a warm, hospitable and relaxing environment, one that is conducive towards enhancing the emotional experience of patients and staff alike. People I have spoken to, who have not visited or resided in hospital as a patient, sometimes react with incredulity when I explain that the interior does not remotely resemble the inside of "the asylum" as depicted in the film One Flew Over The Cuckoo's Nest.

Sticks and Stones

Unfortunately the media has deliberately or
unwittingly (as a result of ignorance) reinforced
negative stereotypes. This can and does make
my work more difficult when speaking to young
children and redressing the imbalance.

Sticks and Stones

(20/2/06 – Evening Gazette)

In previous articles I have highlighted the stigma surrounding mental illness, the myths that perpetuate social exclusions of the mentally ill and the importance of a positive emotional experience of using mental health services. Brick by brick, the wall of discrimination and criminalisation is being pulled down, and modern day mental health services now focus on person-centred care and empowerment of patients to influence care delivery. De-stigmatising mental illness is a passion of mine and over the past four years I have devoted more time to this campaign. I have visited many schools and colleges to spread the word and de-mystify our services. During this period I have been fortunate to have met many wonderful children and supportive teachers all eager to learn about mental illness and its impact on patients and families.

The children I have spoken to have been very receptive with the younger pupils, displaying a maturity far beyond their youth. The children's compassion and non-judgemental attitudes have been very refreshing, contrasting sharply with the often negative stereotyping behaviour of many adults.

Bullying is often raised as a result of the detrimental impact this has on a child's mental health.

Sticks and Stones

Low self-esteem with damaged confidence combine to leave a bullied child feeling totally alone, beyond despair and unsure as to where to turn for help.

Whilst it is encouraging to see schools addressing the problem of bullying more openly, it seems to have reached almost epidemic levels, with increased newspaper headlines devoted to self-harm incidents and the occasional suicide relating a depressing story.

To coincide with world mental health week I was invited to speak to a class of primary school pupils in Hartlepool. I was to spend two hours covering a wide range of mental health issues. In response to asking if anyone in the class had personally experienced bullying, a young girl raised her hand. The class listened intently whilst this young girl disclosed the details of the bullying and how this made her feel, at the time and now.

A number of pupils shuffled nervously in their seats as the young girl recounted the distress and emotional pain she had endured while myself and others in the room were all touched by her courage and determination to tell her story.

It was a poignant moment for all concerned and one that I will never forget. In contrast some school sessions are more light-hearted, where humour is used to break down barriers and develop a rapport.

Sticks and Stones

Stringent measures to tackle bullying have been made in many schools, bullying charters being one example. Mental health awareness in schools is an area that will receive more government funding as part of future planning of healthcare services.

I will continue my input to tackle the stigma and raise awareness within schools as clearly more work still needs to be done in this area. In the meantime, I am grateful to the teachers who have opened their classrooms and minds to me, and the little girl who stood up, alone, to tell her story.

Sticks and Stones

(8/5/06 – Evening Gazette)

SINCE writing this column I have been overwhelmed by the number of people who have approached me to say they have read it, and are in agreement with the message I am trying to deliver.

It is particularly rewarding when I am approached by patients who express gratitude and appreciation that the message is finally being heard. It is one that is long overdue, and hopefully now people are less inclined to judge or stigmatise the mentally ill.

Some of these patients experience discrimination almost on a daily basis in areas such as housing, employment, healthcare and the criminal justice system.

Only by highlighting this discrimination can we tackle the inequality that exists. The media play a crucial role in positively promoting mental health and not jumping on the bandwagon of negatively reinforcing stereotypes.

Recently I attended the first SHIFT international conference in Manchester on stigma and discrimination in mental health. It was extremely informative and particularly emotive because some of the speakers at the conference experience mental health problems themselves, or are carers of a person with a mental illness.

Sticks and Stones

One lady likened the impact of being stigmatised and socially excluded to death by a thousand pin pricks. As a consequence of her husband having a mental illness she found herself and her husband ostracised by her village community, whereas previously they had been very active in the local community with such events as the village fete. Now they found themselves socially rejected.

It was a remark that was made at a party when she had offered her husband as a helper at the local village hall that she was told "but he's a nutter isn't he? We cannot have him helping, what would other people think?".

Stigma is often much worse than the illness itself and once someone has recovered from a mental illness - and yes many people do recover - then the stigma remains. Another example of ignorance was recounted by a lady who was a qualified teacher. Unfortunately this lady had experienced depression and following a seven-year absence from work felt that the time was right to return to another form of work that involved supervising others.

Following her interview this lady was encouraged to study for a GCSE in light of her mental health problems, which came as a bit of a shock to her as she already had a degree and her intellect was not impaired.

Sticks and Stones

We need to look beyond the label, we need to respect the different qualities people possess and not be so judgemental. There is no doubt many others who have experienced the same discrimination and ignorance do not have the opportunity to tell their story and may not have the support of family or friends.

These are the silent victims who deal with their pain and social isolation on a daily basis. It is because of this that the work I carry out, along with others like me, needs to continue.

Sticks and Stones

(24/8/06 – Evening Gazette)

I went with my colleague, Marjorie Wilson, to the Redcar and Cleveland Primary School Conference at the Eston and City Learning Centre.

It focused on the social and emotional aspects of learning (SEALS) and our involvement was to promote an anti-bullying initiative called Story Sacks.

Story Sacks is an approach that raises awareness of the detrimental impact of bullying on a child's emotional health and well-being through storytelling and a book review.

The programme we aim to promote within primary schools is based on the book "The Huge Bag of Worries" by Virginia Ironside. Each session will give children an insight into understanding emotional heath and well-being, the implications of not dealing with problems, and increased understanding of the effect that bullying can have on someone's emotional health.

It is interactive and designed to capture the child's imagination as well as deliver a serious message through play. Marjorie and myself were invited to pilot this programme at Ravensworth Junior School and this proved to be very successful. The day ended with a release of balloons in the playground, with each balloon representing a worry that the child could let go of. Personally, I

Sticks and Stones

see this programme as a creative idea that will further de-stigmatize mental health. Children often find themselves victims of bullying, they cannot always articulate their fears and worries.

Our input will reinforce to pupils and teachers alike the importance of sharing worries, not suffering in silence, and of protecting our emotional health and well-being. A story I was recently told involved a young girl who was being bullied at school. This young girl did not feel able to share her worries with her friends or parents. Instead she would sit on the end of her bed each evening and talk to the only trusted friend she thought she had, her pet dog. If the work we aim to carry out in primary schools goes some way to prevent this kind of situation happening it will have been a success.

Early indications following the conference show a positive response to our programme. Our trust's Passionate People campaign will continue to visit schools and colleges to tackle stigma and discrimination surrounding mental health.

There is still a long way to go.

Sticks and Stones

(20/11/06 – Evening Gazette)

Recently on a training day in Manchester I met a gentleman who impressed me greatly. David has an illness labelled Bipolar Affective Disorder which is characterised by extreme mood swings.

On occasions David's behaviour can be very excitable and sometimes bizarre. Often sufferers from this type of mental illness have found themselves misunderstood and stigmatised by others.

David informed me that this is not the case where he lives and his friends and neighbours accept him for who he is. They look beyond the label and see the person, not the illness. This means a great deal to David and many like him.

David has warmth, a good sense of humour and an engaging charisma. It is easy to see why he is so popular in his local area.

David told me that after many years he had finally come to terms with his illness and does not allow it to disrupt his day to day living too much. He also challenges those who would seek to ridicule or ostracise him for being "different" when exhibiting bizarre behaviour. David described to me his acceptance of his condition in a broad Mancunian dialect, occasionally interlacing the points he was making with witty asides.

Sticks and Stones

He spoke candidly about his traumatic childhood which was deprived of love, affection and family stability, so important in shaping our lives in later years.

It is because of this that he now appreciates the unconditional support of his friends and neighbours as he confronts the daily challenges of his mental illness.

David is not only a survivor he is also an inspiration to others, including myself.

Sticks and Stones

(19/2/07 – Evening Gazette)

A new Department of Health initiative, Action on Stigma, aims to reduce the stigma and discrimination towards those who experience mental illness in the workplace.

I and many others wholeheartedly welcome this approach. This is a positive step forward in creating better understanding and recognition of the vulnerability of all of us, and the way we can support each other in times of need.

The aim of Action on Stigma is to foster a more caring, non-judgemental and empathic culture within the workplace, one where people do not feel stigmatised by openly admitting they are experiencing stress, or any other mental health condition.

People use a variety of reasons to explain their absence. They often avoid stress related illness as a reason because of the associated stigma, and the perceived reaction of managers and colleagues. Ignorance breeds ignorance, and the common misconceptions and negative stereotypes only perpetuate this belief.

Through this initiative six principles will be outlined. These will focus on staff awareness of mental health symptoms, the importance of looking after our mental health, warning signs to look out for, and access to the appropriate help available.

From a mental health clinician's viewpoint I see this initiative as long overdue and hope it will reduce further the discrimination people with mental health problems have experienced, and still do experience, in the workplace.

We all have a responsibility as a caring and compassionate society to embrace these changes. One in six of the population suffer from a mental illness at some time in their lives. Of those 90% want to work. Unfortunately our culture and systems do not always encourage this.

The fear remains of victimisation once in work if an already ignorant culture exists around mental health. This initiative will hopefully remove the discrimination and ignorance once and for all.

Our "Story Sacks" work in primary schools emphasising the importance of sharing worries and concerns continues.

This is highlighting our emotional health and well-being needs, and what we can all do to protect these. The focus is on bullying, which can seriously damage a child's self esteem and confidence.

The teachers have welcomed our input. This complements the important work they carry out in

Sticks and Stones

relation to addressing the emotional needs of the children. Our project is still in the pilot stage and the early indications are promising. Our school input also allows us the opportunity to speak to the teachers about general mental health issues, and maybe alter some misconceptions that exist about our services.

In one of our recent visits to my native East Cleveland the response of the children at Handale Primary School in Loftus impressed me greatly. They asked many questions, some of these showing a maturity beyond their years.

Two examples being "What is bipolar affective illness?" and "How do drugs and alcohol affect your mental health?". These type of questions are generally asked in the comprehensive and college educational setting.

Today's child is tomorrow's adult. Equipping these youngsters now with the knowledge and understanding of mental health will help establish a more compassionate, non-discriminatory society in the future. Maybe we as adults could learn from our children?

When talking to the children I have often seen in their small faces a look of compassion, and an eagerness to understand. This being in sharp contrast to the remarks and behaviour from some adults.

Sticks and Stones

A lesson I have learnt during my school visits is never to underestimate our children, and the children in this region are a shining example to us all.

Sticks and Stones

(16/10/07 – Evening Gazette)

The media play a critical role in ensuring the fair coverage of any news issues, none more so I feel, than mental illness.

It is so important when considering any coverage be it on TV, radio, or television, that the correct message is given.

Sadly this isn't always the case when the focus is on mental illness. People experiencing mental health problems often find themselves unfairly treated by the media. This is often down to ignorance of the facts, but may also be due to a desire to sensationalise stories in order to appeal to a wider audience.

We are all too familiar with headlines such as 'maniac' or 'lunatic' when touching on subjects that people find incomprehensible, such as rape and murder.

Of course, statistically, someone with a mental illness is more likely to be a victim of crime rather than the perpetrator. A few weeks ago I was horrified to read in a popular national newspaper a comment by a reader comparing mental illness to paedophilia, surprisingly stating that those who are mentally ill should be locked up and the key thrown away. This reader's frightening lack of awareness and understanding is again likely to be

Sticks and Stones

the result of biased reporting and wild distortion of the facts.

When I responded to the letter I found my own letter wasn't printed. It would appear that the more controversial the letters are the better. Why let the truth get in the way of a good story, as the saying goes?

So our battle continues and this is a battle between the truth and blatant lies and misinformation. The government is now acknowledging the important role of positively promoting mental health as much as physical health. Money is being invested in programmes all over the country to fight stigma and promote more understanding and respect.

I have recently been funded through the Healthy Communities Programme to raise awareness of mental health issues in the workplace, and challenge the stigma of mental illness within employment. This will be an opportunity to engage with employers and employees to promote acceptance, understanding and support in the workplace for those who experience mental health difficulties.

We will continue to develop our story sacks Huge Bag of Worries project which was delivered to 13 schools within Redcar and Cleveland over the past year. This focuses on supporting the emotional health and well-being of primary school

Sticks and Stones

pupils, and reinforces how bullying damages a child's self confidence and esteem. Our interactive programme has received very positive feedback and evaluation.

Our most recent school visit was to St Margaret Clitherows Primary School in South Bank, where we received a very warm welcome by the teachers and the pupils. It is so uplifting to see the children and teachers respond in such a positive manner to our input. We were particularly touched by the affection of the children, and as always our helium balloon release at the end of the day in the playground went down a treat.

We are now exploring ways in which we can adapt this simple idea for an older audience, particularly the Year 7 pupils in comprehensive schools. This is a difficult year for the pupils with the transition between a primary and comprehensive setting.

Again, we will look at the emotional needs of the children and de-stigmatize our mental health services as before. I also view this as an opportunity to engage with the teachers to support the important work they already do.

Sticks and Stones

(11 March 2008 – Evening Gazette)

Loony, psycho, maniac. These are labels used by some people when belittling people with mental health problems either in jest or with the intention of insulting and offending. Though I would imagine if the shoe was on the other foot, so to speak, we wouldn't really appreciate being called these names ourselves would we?

Maybe we use these derogatory terms as a defence for our own insecurities? If we can belittle someone else and therefore deflect attention away from ourselves we may feel more secure about ourselves. Whatever the rhyme or reason, it is still worth considering why we insist on the use of language that is demeaning, and would it not be better to be more sensitive to the impact certain words can have on a person's self-worth and esteem?

They say sticks and stones may break my bones but words will never hurt me, but I doubt that is really the case. Unless of course there are some people reading this who have never felt hurt through name calling, particularly as a child. Unlikely, I would think.

It becomes almost a second language to some to use such demeaning words when relating to someone perceived as different to ourselves. Or we endeavour to make people laugh by using

Sticks and Stones

words such as those listed above, thinly disguised as humour. Hilarious, I think not.

Particularly if you happen to find yourself on the receiving end. A person standing at a bus stop or walking down the street may become an easy target for those intent on amusing their friends with the odd jibe. And sadly it is not only children we are talking about here. All because that person may have different mannerisms or facial expressions that draw attention to them.
Where do we start to address and challenge this behaviour? We start in primary school and hope that the parents will reinforce the message of tolerance and understanding within the home environment.

If we can de-stigmatize mental illness at an early stage in the child's development, such as in primary school, it is hoped the children we are reaching become better informed, more understanding, and more accepting of other people's differences- normalising rather than mystifying the process of mental health.

Nobody would point their finger at someone in the street, laugh, and remark that that person is a diabetic. So why do we do that to someone with schizophrenia?

Interestingly, we can laugh and even boast about bizarre behaviour often exhibited when heavily drunk because this is what being young is all

Sticks and Stones

about. Quite often it is acknowledged as the inevitable consequence of "a good night out." And yet when we observe someone who is sober, but may be responding to voices due to being mentally ill, we find this less comfortable to come to terms with. We struggle to accept this behaviour as being a socially acceptable norm.

Racism and homophobic language and behaviour is outlawed universally.

We have become a fairer and more tolerant society and we now celebrate our diversity. However, when relating to mental illness it is still deemed to be socially acceptable to use certain types of negative descriptive language, language that would not be tolerated if targeted at other discriminated sections of society.

My work is all about promoting more tolerance and understanding. It is about encouraging more social inclusion for those who experience mental illness, of whom many often find themselves socially excluded. This isn't because it is something I have been asked to so, or I am doing under duress. It is something that I believe in.

Promoting social inclusion isn't just about ticking boxes to confirm a section of society, in my case the mentally ill, have had their rights acknowledged, so job done. A paper exercise it isn't. No, it is about believing people have a right to be entitled to equality in everything. An equal

Sticks and Stones

footing, a level playing field, whether this is in relation to healthcare, employment, housing or the criminal justice system; all of these areas where discrimination against the mentally ill occurs at an unacceptable level.

Despite one in six of the population experiencing mental illness at some point in their lives, many of us believe "it will never be me."
And so we have created a society of "them" and "us" with "us" being the lucky ones.

Sticks and Stones

(14 May 2008 - – Evening Gazette)

Recently on holiday in Ireland we found ourselves in the local Indian Restaurant having a meal. My eyes were drawn towards a man sat in the entrance of the restaurant who was clearly experiencing auditory hallucinations, or in more lay person's terms, "hearing voices". He was periodically shouting obscenities and every now and again a female member of staff would walk over and sit beside him. He would shout and swear when looking in her direction, and also indiscriminately towards those who were either entering or leaving the restaurant. Or so it seemed. On closer observation he was in fact responding to the voices he was hearing and his anger was directed at the voices from wherever they came, not the people in the vicinity.

Most people walked past unaffected by his outbursts, and, as they say in Ireland "passed no remarks" to either him or the member of staff he was sat with. For me as a mental health nurse the sight of someone openly responding to voices was nothing out of the ordinary, having spent many years working within psychiatric hospitals. This would have been a much more common sight many years ago when medication and treatment wasn't as effective as it is now in controlling auditory hallucinations.

After a while the man stopped shouting and at this point the female member of staff brought out a meal for him to eat at the table. The lady wasn't in the least bit intimidated by his outbursts. In fact she looked very composed and relaxed.

Hearing voices can be a disturbing experience for the person who hears them, and also others, such as close family and friends. If the voices are making derogatory remarks and are relentlessly critical, the person experiencing them may feel worn down and extremely upset by their intrusive nature. Fortunately medication is now much more effective in the treatment of auditory hallucinations, and in many cases will eradicate them completely. This will help the person to lead as normal a life as possible, with the feeling that they have a degree of control over the symptoms.

Psychological approaches, such as Cognitive Behavioural Therapy, can teach different coping strategies to help the person understand their personal experiences of "hearing voices" and adapt their lifestyle to deal with them.

Schizophrenia is the condition commonly associated with hearing voices, though stress, excessive alcohol, drug misuse, and brain injury can all result in a person hearing voices. It is much more common than many think.

There are also cultural variations when looking at the experience of hearing voices. Western culture usually equates voices with symptoms of mental illness, therefore often when someone "admits" to

Sticks and Stones

hearing voices the stigma of having a mental illness is further perpetuated. Other cultures regard hearing voices as a spiritual experience, a special gift that one possesses, rather than an illness to be cured.

Some people may find hearing voices quite comforting, and the language content complimentary. Hearing voices can then be interpreted as a positive aspect of their lives. Often the stigma associated with hearing voices prevents people from openly accepting that they do hear voices. As a consequence they then deny themselves the benefit of medication or counselling to treat them.

The man in the restaurant clearly wasn't hearing complimentary voices as he appeared agitated and upset. I was impressed with the attitude of those who decided to ignore his abuse, therefore not agitating him even more by overreacting, and the member of staff who sat with him quietly reassuring him in a calm, relaxed manner. This man was obviously local and the reaction of those in the restaurant gave out the message of "It's okay, there's no need to be alarmed, we've seen it all before." In many ways this is normalising the whole experience, and goes a long way towards encouraging more acceptance and understanding of someone else's differences. What I observed was social acceptance and also social inclusion, these not just being politically correct slogans, but a visible display of genuine compassion and

Sticks and Stones

tenderness.

This man posed no threat to anybody. To some he may have been perceived to be the aggressor because of his shouting and swearing, but in my eyes he was the victim of his own mind. If anything he was frightened and responded positively to reassurance and empathy. Nothing more was required.

I observed with admiration the therapeutic way in which the whole situation was carefully managed, without undue alarm or panic. At no point did I feel threatened, and it was clear to me that others in the vicinity didn't either. Non more so than the staff member who openly engaged with the man and eventually calmed him down in a softly spoken, reassuring voice. Few words were exchanged between the man and the member of staff but I could measure his gratitude through his eye contact, which spoke volumes. I and others present that night would have probably felt more intimidated and threatened in a busy town centre on a Saturday night surrounded by people who are drunk, aggressive, and looking for a fight. After all this man was ill, what would their excuses be?

Sticks and Stones

(August 2008 – Evening Gazette)

"Pull yourself together!" is that often used phrase when speaking to someone who suffers from depression and is struggling to cope. It probably says more about the person uttering it than the intended recipient. The person may feel totally helpless themselves in dealing with the situation and to alleviate this sense of "helplessness" tries to spur the person on to instant recovery, problem solved – if only it was that simple.

Depression is an illness that comes in many shapes and forms, but also has a commonality of symptoms. Low mood, lack of energy and drive, negative thoughts about oneself and the world around, and feeling completely overwhelmed by everything are just a few. Now try "pulling yourself together" out of that little list. People can become over emotional and sometimes have thoughts that scare them, such as "is it all worth it?" and "others would be better off without me". Nightmarish thoughts, but real all the same, painfully real to the person experiencing them.

The depressed person may find that their appetite has decreased, or gone completely, they cannot sleep as negative thoughts take control. As frightening and negative thoughts completely dominate their thinking they struggle to climb out of bed and face the next day. The next day arrives with a multitude of stresses the world and his dog

Sticks and Stones

have brought along to throw at them. Seemingly insignificant daily tasks become unbearable events to face up to, exaggerated beyond reason or rationale, and the world seems like a dark place where there is no escape. Throw in the occasional panic attack for good measure and you have all the ingredients of a nice cake of despair.

And there's more! A person may find themselves overeating, "comfort eating ," and sleep for too long, or may not even have the motivation to get out of bed at all. The less you do the less you want to do, and that leaves the person feeling totally lethargic. These are just a few of the often incapacitating symptoms of depression, and the list goes on. The task of pulling oneself together immediately is nigh impossible, and if anything it places more unnecessary pressure on the sufferer to be what they cannot be, and do what is beyond them at the time. It isn't helpful at all.

Depression, as with any other mental illness, is not something one would like to experience if given the choice. Choices in the matter we do not always have, they are a luxury many can ill afford. So it is important when faced with these symptoms that a person acknowledges their own experiences, and doesn't try to mask or deny what they are going through. All too often the stigma surrounding mental illness makes people think twice about accepting that they have a problem, and as a consequence they somehow perceive themselves to be weak, and less able than others.

Sticks and Stones

Acceptance is the first step to help and the road to recovery.

It is also imperative that other people are more considerate and aware of their own attitudes and opinions. Words can be very powerful weapons used against someone who is struggling to cope, when their self esteem cannot sink any lower. Even if they are spoken in desperation and not with the intention to cause upset, it can backfire.

Depression doesn't discriminate; it respects no social, religious or cultural boundaries and can equally affect both men and women. Young men in particular are at risk because of their difficulty in "opening up" and talking about their feelings, and peer pressure doesn't help. My message to men in particular is simple; do not feel that you are any less of a man because you are experiencing depression, or stress, or whatever word you would like to use to describe your plight. The symptoms are the same for both men and women.

If anyone experiences these kind of symptoms it is a warning sign that must be heeded, in particular the negative thoughts. Listen to what your mind and body is telling you and seek help. We cannot exist without the help and support of others, be it through friendships or families. It is in times of distress when we feel we are struggling that friends and family support become paramount, and they crucially play a significant role in the treatment of depression and the recovery process.

Sticks and Stones

We all need to feel a sense of belonging, this is normal, and having close social contact will enable this. Medication will greatly help to chemically lift the mood, and counselling also has a part to play if required. Often it is not only one but a number of factors that will help someone to recover from depression. All of the above will give the person suffering a sense of hope and help them to look to the future, once they have accepted there is a future again. The next time you feel at a loss as to what to say in reaction to someone's symptoms and behaviours rather than use the phrase "pull yourself together" say nothing. It will cause less harm to the sufferer, and you will not feel so bad yourself.

Sticks and Stones

"A PERSONAL VIEW OF MENTAL ILLNESS" As told to Moira Crawford in Practice Nurse 6 June 2008

Men may refuse to believe they have mental health problems and fail to seek help - even those you would expect to spot the signs early on, as Lol Butterfield, a senior mental health nurse in Cleveland, can testify. Four years ago, Lol was suffering from stress and depression, which built up over several months, affecting his concentration, mood and sleep. Despite his own psychiatric training, he admits he was probably in denial about the symptoms, and thought he was coping.

"In my profession I come up against stress and depression every day, but I somehow felt I was above it all - it couldn't happen to me – and I effectively stigmatised the condition myself", he recalls. Eventually his manager suggested he take some time off and accept treatment, and after 2 or 3 months he had recovered and was back at work. Interestingly, although other colleagues may also have suspected Lol's problems, no one had said anything, reflecting perhaps that even in that environment it wasn't an issue anyone wanted to broach with someone in a senior position. "Everyone was very welcoming and concerned for me when I returned however, and if we can't be understanding in our profession, then who can be?" said Lol.

Sticks and Stones

The experience has taught Lol some important lessons, too. "It has helped me to understand my own tolerances and recognise the triggers that could set off my stress again" he said. "I have become more insightful about remaining well, and more in control, which keeps me more on top of my own mental health," he continued. "It's been a huge learning curve for me, despite my training as a psychiatric nurse. If I hadn't taken that time off, had counselling and medication, and had instead persevered, I don't think I would have fully recovered. I'd be in a constant state of being not quite well and trying to keep going. I'm better, but it doesn't mean it can't happen again, and I have got to be hyper vigilant and do things to keep myself well."

Lol did not experience any discrimination related to his condition, but he knows of many clients who have had bad experiences of this kind, ranging from careless remarks and laughter and worry about filling out forms that enquire whether the applicant has ever suffered a mental health problem, to outright discrimination, particularly in employment. As a result, he is channelling energy into trying to reduce the stigma of mental illness, and his Trust has allowed him to take a part- time secondment to work in schools and workplaces to raise the profile of mental illness and reduce its stigma.

He has worked on a schools programme entitled The Huge Bag of Worries, which addresses the issues of bullying and reducing the stigma

Sticks and Stones

surrounding mental health problems. In the workplaces he visits he talks to staff and employers about discrimination against people with mental health problems. He also acts as a spokesperson for the Speakers' Bureau, raising the profile of mental health with the media, and writing a regular column in the local paper about mental health.

He agrees that men tend to be less willing than women to talk openly about their health and particularly their mental health, although this is changing. "It is becoming more acceptable to admit what might previously have been considered 'weakness'", he said. Where he works in Cleveland, however, there is a great deal of heavy industry and the accompanying 'macho' culture in which men still try to mask or cover up stress. "It's generally a hard job to get men attending any kind of health awareness raising sessions, but particularly mental health ones," he said, adding: "It might be different in an office environment where people do more talking".

Lol puts the disproportionately high number of suicides among young men down to the continuing shame that they feel about their own condition. "They feel less of a person", he said, "and that no-one else is talking about stress. They have a lack of understanding of their condition and feel they can't talk about it. They lose insight, and it's particularly sad because actually there is more help out there for them then there has ever been".

Sticks and Stones

Much of this perceived stigma possibly comes from the sufferer himself. "People self stigmatize. They expect it from others, and it becomes a self-fulfilling prophecy," he warned. "While there's no doubt that it does sometimes occur, often the level of discrimination and stigma that is out there is far less than the person expects."

Lol blamed the tabloid press for much of the misunderstanding and fear that exists in the public mind about mental health. "Headlines that read "nutter", "psycho" or "maniac" are sensational but in fact 95% of serious crimes are committed by people without mental health problems. That means only 5% are committed by people with mental health problems, which always amazes the people I talk to. We have to educate people to understand that most criminals are bad not mad".

As for whether men might be more likely to open up to a male health professional than a female one, he is doubtful. "My own counsellor was a woman, and I was more than happy to talk to her about my stress and depression", he said. "By and large I"d prefer to talk to a female, but people may tend to assume that women are more understanding, compassionate and caring then men, and less likely to think you are "less of a man" for admitting mental health problems".

His advice to practice nurses on helping men with mental health problems is firstly to "normalise" the problem. "Thank and praise them for confiding in you," he advised, "but don't get out of your depth and be sucked in to acting as a counsellor if you are not trained for it. You could be opening a can of worms." If you believe a person is suffering from stress and/or depression, give them the option of seeing their GP to be offered counselling or medication, or ideally both, he argues. "Try to help them see that mental health is not separate to physical health. They don't need to be any more embarrassed about a problem that is in the mind than a physical illness or injury. A lot of the stigma about mental health is about seeing it as separate from physical health, but they are very closely linked. Physical wellness and exercise keeps us mentally healthy too." Sensitive use of language, tact and discretion are key, he added, to helping a person who feels stigmatized to admit to a problem.

Sticks and Stones

(January 2009-Evening Gazette)

Following my previous article a number of people have approached me and commented on George, a patient I nursed many years ago. They were touched by his particular poignant story. It was one of arrest and torture during the second world war when working as a teacher in Germany. For my part I try to personalise stories such as Georges because it helps the reader to look beyond the 'patient' label and clinical diagnosis to appreciate the real person. Hopefully people can then empathise more by not characterising people by their 'conditions' or 'illnesses' but view them as unique individuals with thoughts and feelings, unique life experiences, and personal qualities we could all learn from.

George had a psychotic illness, schizophrenia, and this was treated mainly by the use of major tranquillisers (phenothiazines) to control his voices (auditory hallucinations) and paranoid thinking (delusions) The medication used also dampened his agitation, this being the result of experiencing such distressing symptoms. The word schizophrenia stems from the Greek words of schizein (to split) and phren (mind) It is though highly misleading when people describe schizophrenia as being a 'split mind'. It is a much more complex and illness and not as simple as that to define.

Sticks and Stones

Georges treatment may have been very different today. Previously the approach would have been one of eliminating the voices he heard. Nowadays alongside conventional medication to try to achieve this a psychological approach aimed at learning to 'live with his voices' might have been adopted. Psychological interventions (talking therapies) were not acknowledged to be as successful then in treating psychosis and were focused more on affective (mood) disorders, such as depression. In the late 1970s and early 1980s the medication used was helpful in as far as controlling the symptoms though often resulted in the patient experiencing many distressing side effects.

Nowadays there are more effective medication treatment outcomes and far less distressing side effects for the patient to experience. Psychiatric treatment programmes have come a long way, but sadly stigmatizing attitudes and opinions remain. Although I would have been optimistic and hopeful of Georges treatment regime today, I would still have concerns about the attitude of others impacting on Georges overall quality of life.

 Following the closure of many large psychiatric hospitals in the late 1980's George and many like him may have struggled to re adapt to living independently in the community, some with far less support than previously. They had spent many years , sometimes a lifetime, living within

Sticks and Stones

the walls of an institution. They had become disempowered, deskilled and dependent on the staff who were tasked with caring for them, such as myself. It was therefore imperative that the planned after care in the community met their individual needs appropriately.

The attitude and behaviour of others towards George once discharged needed to reflect acceptance back into the community, understanding of his situation, and empathy for his condition. George had as much right to be socially accepted and to feel part of society as anyone else. Many would argue that he perhaps had more right than most to acceptance and respect following his capture and torture, considering his subsequent mental illness was a direct consequence of his defence of his country. For that he paid a high price, more than most he paid with his sanity.

I spoke about the acceptance of George by the local community and this meant he felt safe wandering around the town late at night alone and drinking in the local pubs. He was an interesting gentleman who, when mentally well, enjoyed nothing more than to socialise with others. I would often see him sat at the bar entertaining the staff with his much travelled stories and his passion for politics. His idiosyncratic ways would have drawn some unwanted attention to him but to my recollection he never experienced verbal or physical abuse because of this. He became part of the local community and was not ostracised or alienated because he had a mental illness.

The likelihood of George relaxing at the bar today, or wandering alone at night and not finding himself an innocent victim, I would believe unlikely. For whatever reason, or reasons, society appears to be less tolerant these days. Sadly in our daily rush through life the Georges of this world often get left behind if they cannot keep up with the pace.

George was one example. What we often fail to understand, or forget, is that many people who experience mental illness, of whatever kind, live very ordinary and independent lives. Ordinary people who live next door to you and I as teachers, plumbers, mechanics and a wide range of professions, skilled and unskilled. People who live in families and also alone. Their outward physical appearance rarely betrays the fact that they have a mental illness. Being wrapped in bandages, or walking on crutches being the obvious consequence of a physical injury, the mind it is much more subtle and less obvious to read. The different medications, treatment and support they receive at home helps them to lead fulfilling lives, thus enabling them to make positive contributions in society.

If we all view mental health and mental illhealth as a continuum which anyone at any time of their

Sticks and Stones

lives can experience this may go some way towards tackling the stigma aspect. It will certainly remove the them and us belief and the ignorance many unfortunately endorse.

Sticks and Stones

(November 2008-Evening Gazette)

Nearly 30 years ago as a teenager I first set foot in a psychiatric hospital. It was called Fairfield hospital and was an imposing Victorian "asylum" set in nearly 200 acres of rolling countryside in Hertfordshire. I had travelled from the North East to work in the hospital, initially as a porter, before going into mental health nursing. Little was I to know at the time that it was to be the start of a long career in the National Health Service. Even though it was almost 30 years ago I still remember it as if it was yesterday.

My mind was racing with stereotypical images of the patients walking around in a zombie like state, and all exhibiting strange mannerisms. My thinking had been influenced by the countless films I had seen on television and at the cinema, as well as newspaper reports of "loonies" and "maniacs" being incarcerated for the safety of others. I was both excited and apprehensive.

I was pleasantly surprised when I started my new role and I did see patients wandering around the hospital corridors and grounds. Some of whom did display mannerisms that drew unwanted attention to them, but that was as much a consequence of the side effects of the medication they were taking as the symptoms of their illnesses.

Sticks and Stones

But what struck me most was the community spirit, and the bustling day to day lives of staff and patients played out before my very eyes. The long shiny corridors echoed to the sound of feet constantly walking up and down going from one ward or office to another. Outside in the grounds on hot summer days cricket and football would be played and spectators would sit on nearby benches and watch, or just relax.

This scene was far removed from all the preconceived negative thoughts I had imagined of high walls, keeping the 'nutters' safely locked in and guarded by burly men in white coats. The hospital was surrounded by an assortment of trees and bushes. There were no gates restricting entry and everyone could freely walk around the grounds.

I describe it as a community because that was what it was. Each year the hospital held its fete when all the locals from the nearby villages would visit and staff and patients would man stalls. It was important to show the outside world that the hospital functioned as a hospital, not a prison, and a place where everyone regardless of age, sex, creed or religion would receive the treatment they were entitled to. Treatment for an illness any one of us could at some point in our lives experience.

One of the first patients I met was George (not his real name) George was in his seventies and although in the later years of his life he still walked

Sticks and Stones

with a spring in his step. He had been tortured during the Second World War whilst working as a teacher in Germany and had been ordered to put a picture of Hitler on the classroom wall and he refused. His courage and conviction was to cost him dearly, it cost him his mental health for the rest of his life. He was punished severely for showing insubordination and taking a stand. On his return to England he struggled to survive in the 'outside world' and was admitted into a psychiatric hospital. The hospital was to become his home, his world, for the rest of his days. George had difficulty living independently, his mind was in pieces, and his spirit had been broken. He had become a lost soul who spent his remaining days wandering around the hospital grounds trying to make sense of his life. Or sheer existence as it had now become.

George never spoke about his treatment and torture, preferring to chat about cricket and politics, and in particular Margaret Thatcher, the prime minister at the time, whom he despised. He was a staunch socialist and would informally educate me and my colleagues whenever we met him in the corridors or grounds. He still retained a powerful intellect and was prone to angry verbal outbursts when others disagreed with his views. These were never taken personally as George never intended them to be. He was often shabbily dressed and eccentric in his mannerisms.

Sticks and Stones

When I reminisce about George it is with a deep fondness and admiration for a man who had shown incredible strength and bravery. My colleagues and I all warmed to George, it would have been hard for anybody to dislike him. He was an inspiration to us all though this is not how George may have been perceived outside of the hospital where bigotry and ignorance of mental illness reigned. Whenever George left the hospital to go into the local town, which he occasionally did, his appearance and behaviour would invariably have drawn unwanted attention. I would often see him at night walking around the town, always alone and with only his thoughts for company.

Many locals would have remembered George, as I do, as someone who always stopped to talk and pass the time of day, and someone who could entertain with his remarkable intellect, sense of humour, and extensive political knowledge. He had his idiosyncratic ways that may not have appealed to everyone but this is what made George unique.

Others who did not know George and hadn't formed a relationship may have treated him with the same disdain and stigma that many other patients from the hospital experienced at the time. To them George would be identified as 'the patient from the local asylum' His character defined by his illness, ignorance influencing people's perceptions.

Sticks and Stones

It was through meeting George and understanding him more as a unique individual that I began to understand the devastating personal impact of severe mental illness. It taught me to appreciate the importance of looking beyond the 'labels' we all like to use and value the person on the other side.

I make no apologies for remembering George with a warmth and nostalgia. He possessed personal qualities and attributes we could all learn from. His life story was remarkable and traumatic beyond comprehension. As a young man I admired what he had done and was deeply saddened by the situation he had found himself in. None of us could ever have imagined the abuse George suffered at the hands of his captors. He disclosed very little of this and would probably have taken his dark thoughts and memories to his grave. Daily we read newspaper headlines of the thugs who terrorise our streets, feral youths carrying knives, and hoodies roaming estates at night looking for easy prey. People are attacked indiscriminately and often this is because they are perceived to be 'different', as George was. George would probably have been easy prey as he walked alone at night in today's society, simply minding his own business and alone with his thoughts................. how times have changed.

Sticks and Stones

Stress Factor

(May 2 2005 Evening Gazette article.)

A nurse has called for more support in the workplace for people suffering from mental health problems.

Lol Butterfield, Senior Nurse for Tees and North East Yorkshire NHS Trust, said counselling should be offered for all those suffering from conditions such as stress, anxiety and depression.

New research published by the British Medical Journal shows those conditions have overtaken back pain for incapacity benefit claims.

Since 1995, the number of people reporting stress caused or made worse by their work has doubled and common mental disorders are now the leading cause of sickness absence.

Mr Butterfield said industries and professionals should be more aware of mental health problems. "There seems to be a lot more pressure on people at work and it can be a large cause of sickness" he said.

"We need support services such as counselling in the workplace for these people."

Mr Butterfield believes the increase is due to

Sticks and Stones

raised awareness to mental health conditions.

"There was something of a stigma attached to stress and depression. Now more people are willing to acknowledge when they are depressed or stressed."

Statistics from the Department for Work and Pensions show that in August last year 41,200 people were claiming Incapacity Benefit or severe disability allowance in the Tees Valley.

Mental illness affects one in four people nationally.

.

Sticks and Stones

Sticks and Stones

Sticks and Stones

Sticks and Stones